RUNNING FREE
OF INJURIES

RUNNING FREE
OF INJURIES
FROM PAIN TO PERSONAL BEST

PAUL HOBROUGH

BLOOMSBURY

LONDON · OXFORD · NEW YORK · NEW DELHI · SYDNEY

Bloomsbury Sport
An imprint of Bloomsbury Publishing Plc

50 Bedford Square   1385 Broadway
London   New York
WC1B 3DP   NY 10018
UK   USA

www.bloomsbury.com

First published in 2016
© Paul Hobrough, 2016
Photos © Grant Pritchard and Getty Images

British Library Cataloguing-in-Publication Data
A catalogue record for this book is available from the British Library.

Library of Congress Cataloguing-in-Publication data has been applied for.

ISBN: Print: 978-1-4729-1380-7
       ePDF: 978-1-4729-1382-1
       ePub: 978-1-4729-1381-4

10 9 8 7 6 5 4 3 2 1

Typeset in Seravek by seagulls.net
Printed and bound in China by Toppan Leefung Printing.

Bloomsbury Publishing Plc makes every effort to ensure that the papers used in the manufacture of our books are natural, recyclable products made from wood grown in well-managed forests. Our manufacturing processes conform to the environmental regulations of the country of origin.

To find out more about our authors and books visit www.boomsbury.com. Here you will find extracts, author interviews, details of forthcoming events and the option to sign up for our newsletters.

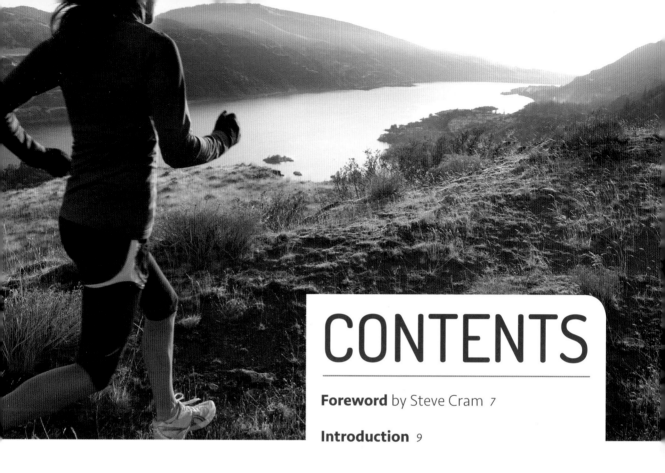

CONTENTS

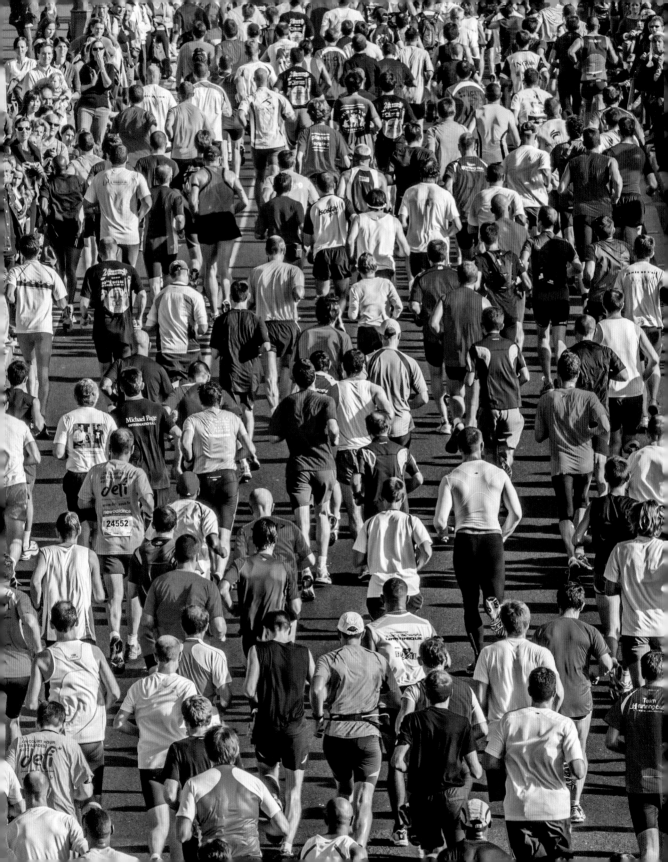

FOREWORD

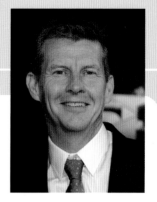

NOW WELL INTO MY FIFTH decade of running, I sometimes think of my body as a classic vintage car. The fast races are a distant memory but I still enjoy the odd spin around the block. Thankfully, all the parts are still there but it needs an expert and caring set of hands and eyes to coax them into action; a top mechanic who understands the thrill of pushing performance, the significance of each tiny component, plus the technology and knowledge to restore and maximize output. That man is Paul Hobrough. I trust my vintage chassis and engine to him, hoping the wheels don't fall off!

I trust him because I can recognize Paul's skill and ability as a physiotherapist. Over my many years as an international athlete and now as a more casual runner and coach to two of Britain's top 1500m runners, I know how rare and important people like Paul are. His energy and enthusiasm are channeled into furthering his own knowledge and experience, which ultimately helps him deliver bespoke and effective interventions and injury management.

As a former world champion and world record holder, I had my fair share of injuries. It is an inevitable part of training and happens to runners of all levels. The key is who and what do you turn to? A good physio needs to be able to quickly recognize the problem, devise the correct treatment protocols and instigate a rehabilitation plan that gets the runner back doing what he or she loves best.

I have met countless physios over the years and while some have been better looking and others more intellectually challenging, Paul is the one who I recommend to friends. We have got to know each other well in recent years, although most of our conversations take place with my face planted well into his physio bed.

Paul has put an immense amount of effort into this book, with an emphasis on case studies from his many satisfied clients. His own experiences as an elite level sportsman and his exposure to others of a similar nature have driven his quest to improve and develop as a physiotherapist. Seminars, courses and hands-on activity have given Paul a comprehensive understanding of his trade with particular relevance to runners.

We are all looking for an easy fix. They rarely exist, but this book will surely give you a great reference to ensure you lose as little time as possible to niggles or more serious injuries.

I thoroughly recommend it to runners of all levels and abilities. This vintage vehicle in particular is hoping to keep on rolling along the roads and with Paul in my pit lane, then I feel confident that it can... even if he occasionally encourages me to oil the wheels a little too much!

Steve Cram

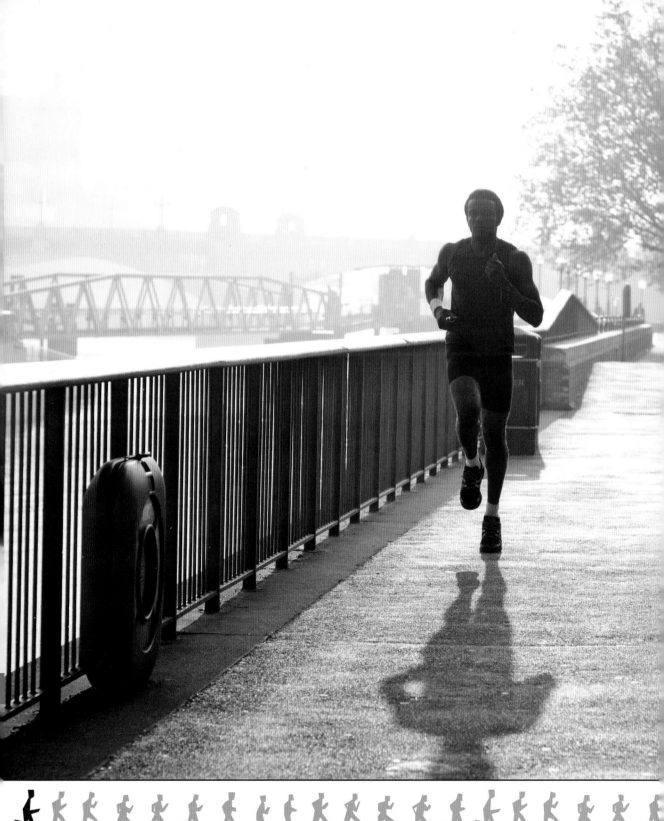

INTRODUCTION

This book has been a long time coming – I've been writing it for years. The reasons for taking such a long time to get pen to paper are threefold: firstly, I considered the subject had been 'done' already by a great many writers, secondly, I see on average 70 clients per week so when am I going to squeeze this in alongside work, three kids, a loving wife and my own training? But lastly and most pertinently, nobody had ever asked me! Writing a book isn't something that many people will ever do and I for one didn't want to take on the challenge with no real chance of anyone ever reading it. The opportunity came when I was commissioned by Bloomsbury Publishing to finally get this book out of my head and onto paper. In short, I would simply have to find the time.

When making a start, I decided upon three goals for the book:

1 I wanted this to be a book that enables you to take it off the shelf at point of injury and learn exactly what to do.
2 I desperately wanted the book to have personality, to get away from a dry, almost surgical read, so expect opinion, sentiment and, at times, effervescence in the text!
3 I have read plenty of scientific journals and also enjoyed the writings of Ben Goldacre in books such as *Bad Science*, but nobody wants me to ramble on too much about research and trials. I believe that you want factual help, safe in the knowledge that the information is bolstered by scientific evidence (and of course referenced properly where necessary).

No science is perfect, a great deal of the stuff we get sold is bad science (so be careful what you read in the papers), but we do need science to tell us right from wrong. Science tells us what happened to a group of participants in a controlled environment and then the results are used to inform the general public of best practice. Ask yourself this though, what similarities are there between you and the twelve American college athletes used as subjects in that piece of scientific research? We have to get information from somewhere, but that somewhere needs to be assessed for validity and evaluated in terms of scientific authority. I ask that you trust the information contained herein has been built up via education both formal (degrees) and informal, passed down from practitioner to practitioner and of course through lots and lots of reading.

I started accumulating knowledge for this book aged 14 when I first walked in to see the osteopath Ron Johnson, in Woking, UK, for significant back pain, which was seemingly going to end my career as a flatwater kayak paddler. He came highly recommended by my coach and three-time Olympian, Eric Jamieson, with tales of miracles performed by this man. That's the thing that happens with a good practitioner, people talk about him or her and therefore marketing is not usually necessary.

I immediately warmed to Ron; he spoke to me directly, involving me in every stage of his deliberations about my back pain. Because I was 14, Ron could have spent the whole time talking to my parents and just treating me without any input on my part, but Ron took the time to involve me in my own therapy, to educate me and to empower me to take control of my own destiny – that was the secret to the success of his treatments. Ron would prescribe me hundreds of exercise repetitions for my back. He did this because he saw an enthusiastic young athlete who felt like his career might be over, but most importantly he knew how to motivate me. He didn't prescribe anything like that to the older woman who came in directly after me; it wouldn't be

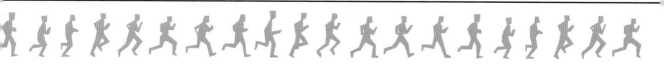

relevant for her. He could see me three times per week; perhaps she came twice a month.

Thanks to Ron, I rehabilitated successfully and, as a result, had a long career as a flatwater kayak paddler, and Ron inspired me to try to do the same for everyone who walks into one of my clinics.

Each individual is treated in an individual way. I want my patients to understand that when I provide them with information, exercises, or treatment, this is specific to them. All too often the patient passes on information personalized for them to another member of their running club, as their friend's injury sounds similar; but this may very well be a mistake. What this book aims to do is to assist you with your own diagnosis, looking at the symptoms and then trying some of the advice contained within the book. Through reading these chapters and increasing your understanding of what to look out for, I hope that you will actually identify injury

FOR PHYSIOS

"In my experience"
"My gut feeling"
"My hunch is" →
"I just know"

Systematic reviews

Randomised controlled trials

Cohort studies

Case control studies

Case series, case reports

Editorials, expert opinion

I'm now into the second decade of my therapeutic career and spend my days working with runners, so I know there is more to helping someone than simply applying the latest 'paint by numbers' scientific fix. For example, in the treatment of an injured ligament, physiotherapists will often use two minutes of deep transverse frictions (DTF) to gain a numbing of the ligament, then ten minutes of the same for therapeutic effect, as has been written down countless times in scientific texts and journals, e.g. how to get the diagnosis and what to do as the treatment programme. Physiotherapy isn't like that though; you can't just diagnose and then provide a card from your folder on the latest rehabilitation protocol. It has to be personalized and there is a great deal of experience behind the diagnosis. The pyramid above will help you to understand some of the philosophy behind the way I reach the diagnosis.

There are some scary statistics for practitioners who choose the exercise card route: only 7% of clients will follow physiotherapy-based exercises to the letter; less than half end up doing just 'some' of the prescribed plan; and a whopping 50% don't do any at all. A patient spends 24 hours a day living with themselves; if they are not going to take on some of the responsibility for their rehabilitation, this leaves a therapist just 30 minutes each week to fix a problem.

The role of the good therapist is to motivate, engage and educate the patient, to drive that 7% closer to 75% and to provide a treatment package that is both personalized and relevant to the end user.

This requires experience and taking the time to understand your client.

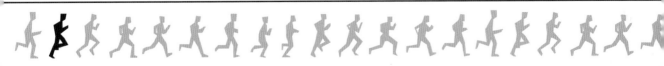

before it starts and therefore run free of injury and obtain that elusive PB.

My early experiences as a patient have shaped the way I work today. I didn't want to be told to come back week after week without good reason, and I wanted to be helped to understand what was wrong and what was going to help fix me. Above all, I wanted to see 'the best', someone who was the leading expert in their field and enjoyed a reputation just like Ron Johnson. If I have even come close to fulfilling these ideals, then I am very proud, though I continue to work hard towards these goals every day. I am a practising physiotherapist to real people in real clinics fulfilling my dream.

So who am I? I have more than one degree to my name (exercise physiology, physiotherapy and the odd postgrad to make up the numbers) but I am not an academic. I am rubbish at general knowledge – but I really like providing the art, or skill, or calling, that is physiotherapy. I cannot claim much more, though I have put my healing hands on the likes of Mo Farah, Steve Cram, Paula Radcliffe, Marilyn Okoro, Allison Curbishley, Scott Overall, Rossco Murray and Laura Weightman, all of whom are Olympians and known to you as a runner (I sincerely hope). If this makes me a good physio in your eyes, then great, but I want to be judged by my clients much more than anyone else.

So my aim was to write a certain number of words a day for 70 successive days. This was my goal: 70,000-odd words and the rest is all pictures. I like goals; they have a tendency of delivering results faster than dreams. I hope this book will ensure that you do the same – set yourself the goal of becoming injury-free.

How the book works

So, onto business. This book starts at the foot and works upwards to the lower back. The aim is to focus on the most common running injuries in the light of scientific research and my own clinical experience. The most common injuries for a runner are:

- Medial tibia stress syndrome (shin splints)
- Achilles tendinopathy
- Plantar fasciitis (heel pain)
- Patellofemoral syndrome (Runner's Knee) (Dias Lopes *et al.*, 2012)

However, I've included many more as I believe that, as is the case with my many clients, you will not conform to what science tells us is the 'norm'.

For each body part discussed in this book, there is a diagram of the area for reference (avoiding footnotes or lengthy explanations of anatomical names), along with the most common injuries that I see in clinic, how to spot them early, how to self-treat them, what to expect from a good physiotherapist and how best to get back into a running regime. Additionally, there are stories from some of my clients about their own personal journey

CROSS TRAINING

This is something that some people consider is only part of your training when you are injured. It is true that you may well spend more of your time cross training when injury strikes but a good programme should be underpinned by additional cross training, be it in strength and conditioning in the gym, or using body weight and stretches, aqua jogging, using the cross trainer, or riding your bike. When injured, seek out exercises that enable you to replicate your aerobic and anaerobic training sessions and do these either in the pool, on the bike, or on the cross trainer. Being injured doesn't mean training has to stop, it just means that you need to get your heart and lungs working using different methods.

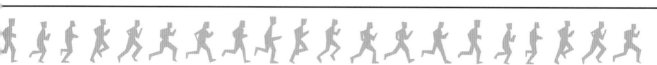

through injury and some examples of training schedules for you to follow.

There will also be exercises for you to do. This is standard physio practice – they really work – but these are cross-referenced firstly as a week-long 'prehab' strategy to keep you pain- and injury-free, and secondly as part of the rehabilitation exercises for each injury. Due to the significant crossover of exercises, these are all clearly referenced at the back of the book, both as a complete list, with picture and bulleted technique points, and also grouped in the index for each exercise to make life easier for you.

Ice versus Heat

First, a quick note about ice and heat. There is a debate raging over what should be applied for acute through to chronic injury. Long-held advice has been to use the Rest, Ice, Compression and Elevation (R.I.C.E.) protocol for acute injury. At this time there is conflicting evidence with more and more research showing that heat can be at least as, if not more, effective than ice in the management of injury and for that matter recovery from exercise (Malanga *et al.*, 2015). Ice has always been seen as the answer to acute injury, owing to the vasoconstriction (narrowing) of vessels bringing unwanted inflammation to the area it causes. It is difficult to see how heat, which is a vasodilator (opening blood vessels) can do the same. The benefits of heat are currently being researched, as is the claim that ice could actually cause more scarring and therefore prolong healing times (Tiidus 2015, Carter, 2015).

For the purpose of this book, I will continue to mention R.I.C.E. in terms of acute injury, however, the continued belief that this remains the best policy is under review. I for one will be continuing my quest for the answers, scanning the literature as it comes to public attention and hope that you will do the same and afford me some latitude on this topic as scientific opinion changes.

There is also a debate regarding non-steroidal anti-inflammatory medicines (NSAIDS) such as ibuprofen. It is believed by some that using these within the first 72 hours after an injury distorts the natural healing process and they should not be taken: does this add weight to the argument in favour of heat rather than ice? One study was unable to find any evidence to support using NSAIDS over paracetamol for pain relief following acute injury (Jones *et al.*, 2015), so perhaps in the light of this evidence we should abandon ibuprofen and the like and be more circumspect in the use of ice for acute injury.

Prehabilitation

Before we get started, let's look at the key exercises for runners to perform weekly as part of a robust 'prehabilitation' programme – what to do if you want to stay as injury-free as possible – through some easy-to-follow, quick exercises. Prehabilitation, or 'prehab' is also known as strength and conditioning (S&C). S&C conjures up images of someone spending 90 minutes in a gruelling gym session, which would be the case for most elite runners, however, it starts with some basic body work exercises, the most valuable of which are detailed here as weekly must-haves for runners.

Prehab is different to a warm-up or a cool down; although there will be some obvious crossovers, the objectives for each are different. A warm-up is, as it sounds, to warm up the body and prepare it for the coming exercise regime; a cool down is used to slowly reduce the heart rate, lengthen soft tissues and speed recovery. What prehab, warm-up and cool down all have in common is their goal of reducing injury. A full warm-up and cool down regimen is included in appendix 2 and appendix 3 respectively.

Starting at the foot, the exercise schedule that follows demonstrates the regime in pictures and with technical pointers, although as with all instructions, be it for flat-pack furniture assembly or learning any new skill, there can be some elements lost in translation.

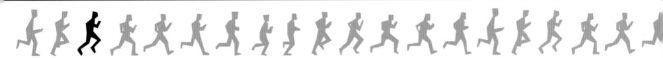

When I put this initial list together, I very quickly listed about 50 key exercises covering strength and flexibility. In physiotherapy we have the same numbers game to play in terms of testing as part of the diagnosis for an injury, as we have numerous tests on offer. The trick is to be able to decide what you 'must' do, what you 'should' do and in the event of having more time, what you 'could' do.

For prehab, there are 21 essential exercises. Other common stretches or exercises, such as a basic hamstring or quad stretch, which might be specific to your injury, will be referred to as part of the rehab programme in each section. For now, let's look at the exercises most people won't be doing already, or may not have heard of before and therefore might provide the greatest positive impact on your ability as a runner, let alone making you more impervious to injury.

Where possible, the exercises chosen have incorporated several muscle areas to be worked simultaneously in an attempt to limit the number of individual exercises and thus the time taken.

It is of course unreasonable to do all 21 exercises each day, therefore the following programme for your week makes it possible to achieve everything noted here on a weekly basis, taking fewer than 12 minutes per day. The full description and recomended length of stretch or number of repetitions can be found in Appendix 1 on pages 167-179.

	Exercises	Time for Prehab (min)
Monday	Core muscles (strength), Hamstring/core combination (strength), Hamstring (stretch), Single leg balance, Soleus (stretch)	10.5
Tuesday	Hip flexors (stretch), Tibialis posterior (strength), Glute activation (strength), Shin (stretch)	10
Wednesday	Single leg squat (strength), Calf raises (strength), Towel grabbing (strength), Hip adductors (stretch)	8.5
Thursday	The clam – hip abduction/rotation (strength), Toe raises (strength), Hamstrings (strength)	10
Friday	Side step with squat (strength), Peroneals – ankle eversion (strength), Single leg squat (strength)	10
Saturday	Calf (stretch), Glutes (stretch), ITB Tensor fascia latae (stretch), Single leg balance, Glute activation (strength)	10
Sunday	Day off prehab	

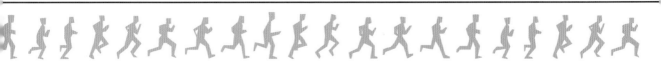

Prehab Exercises

1. Towel grabbing
(STRENGTH) (2 MIN) PAGE 167

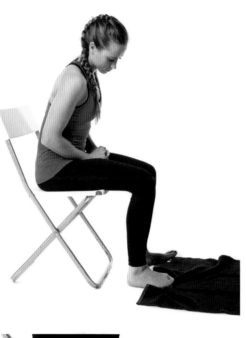

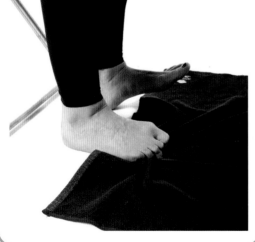

2. Calf
(STRETCH) (1.5 MIN) PAGE 168

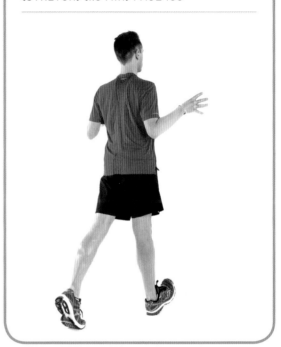

STATIC & DYNAMIC

A static stretch as part of your prehab is still very relevant, although dynamic stretching as part of a warm-up is now favoured. Static stretching is where you place the muscle under tension and hold that position for a period of time; dynamic stretching is increasing the range of movement through a series of repeated movements.

3. Soleus

(STRETCH) (1.5 MIN) PAGE 168

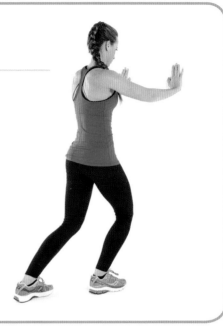

4. Calf raise

(STRENGTH) (3 MIN) PAGE 169

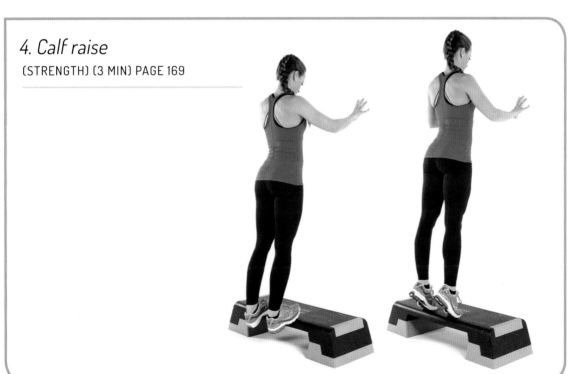

5. Toe raises

(STRENGTH) (3 MIN) PAGE 169

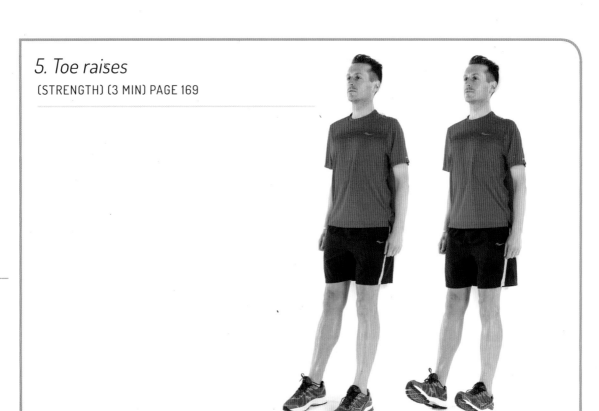

6. Tibialis posterior

(STRENGTH) (3 MIN) PAGE 170

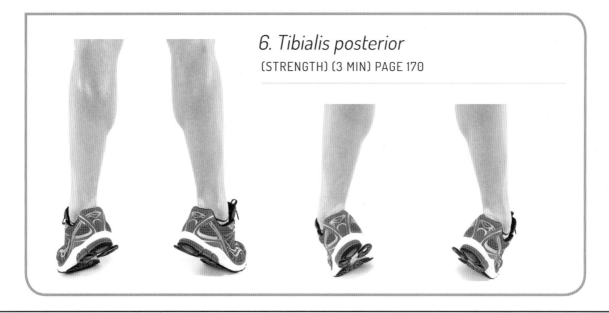

7. Peroneal–ankle eversion
(STRENGTH) (4 MIN) PAGE 170

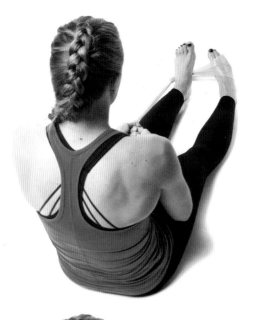

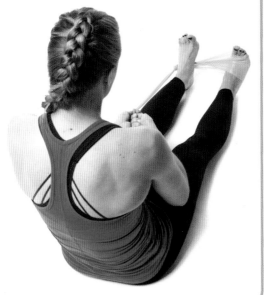

8. Shin
(STRETCH) (1 MIN) PAGE 171

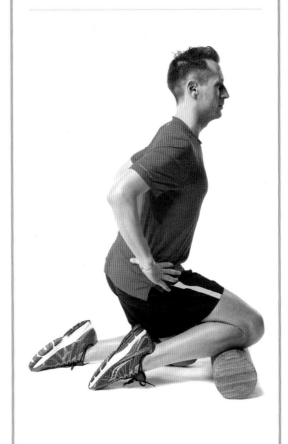

FOOT AND ANKLE PROPRIOCEPTION (BALANCE/STRENGTH)

Start with balancing on the floor, just standing on one leg for 20 seconds at a time. You can try this while you brush your teeth. Then graduate to a pillow or cushion.

In time you will find this easy, so now try with your eyes closed or in the dark. Suddenly you will feel every synapse of each individual nerve trying to keep you upright and working hard to do so.

Once you have developed good balance, you can move to wobble cushions. Wobble boards were used for a long time, but are really very difficult to master, so the introduction of wobble cushions and BOSU® balls, etc., are making functional training more and more popular. A beneficial bi-product of this new craze of functional training is that people are now working their balance muscles more than ever before and the ankles of the world should rejoice.

9. Single leg balance
(2-4 MIN) PAGE 171

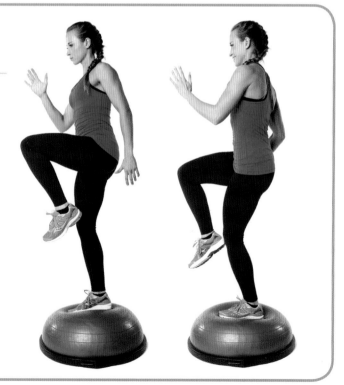

Variations: BOSU® lunge
(4 MIN) PAGE 172

The BOSU® lunge is an extension of the previous exercise and can be used instead of the basic balance once you have attained a suitable level of balance.

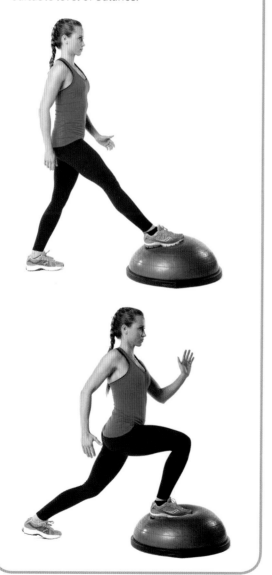

Lunge into single leg balance
(4 MIN) PAGE 172

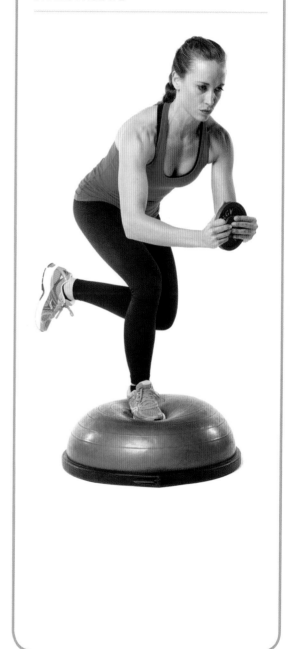

10. The clam – Hip abduction/rotation
(STRENGTH) (4 MIN) PAGE 173

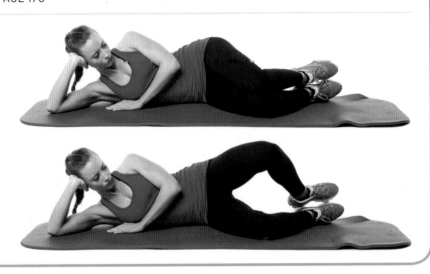

11. Hip flexors
(STRETCH) (1.5 MIN) PAGE 173

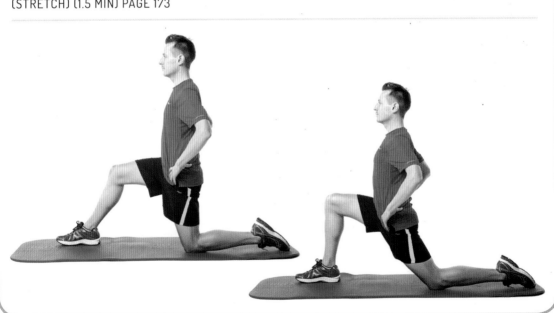

RUNNING FREE OF INJURIES

12. Hip adductors
(STRETCH) (1.5 MIN) PAGE 174

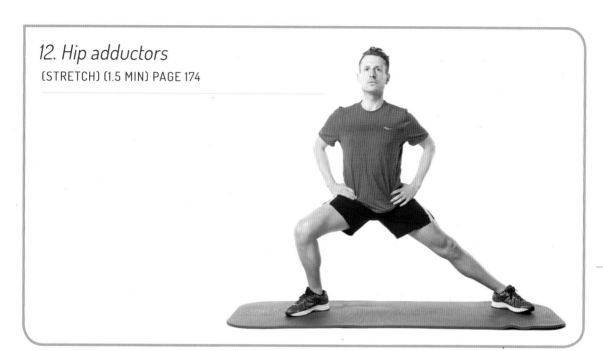

13. Hamstrings
(STRENGTH) (4 MIN) PAGE 174

This exercise has been chosen as it combines lower back strength, hamstring strength, core strength, foot, ankle, knee and hip balance, plus shoulder and upper back stabilization and posture.

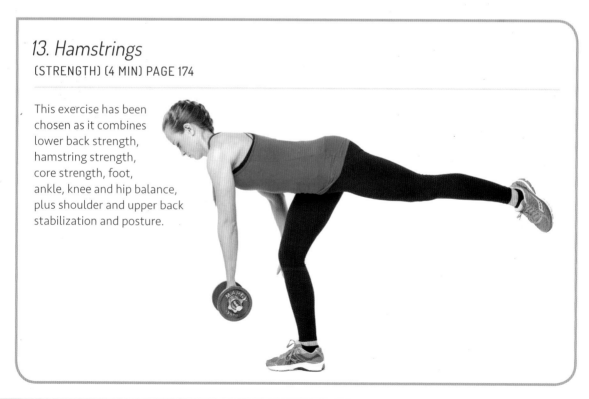

14. Single leg squat
(STRENGTH) (2 MIN) PAGE 175

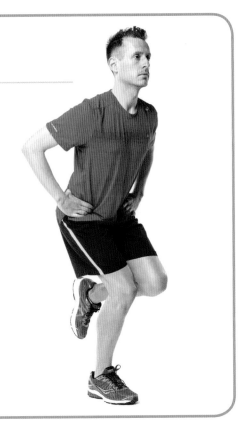

15. Glute activation
(STRENGTH) (4 MIN) PAGE 175

This exercise strengthens the core muscles, in a combination of the plank, glute activation and shoulder stabilization exercises.

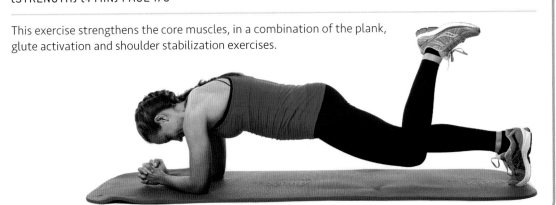

16. Core muscles
(STRENGTH) (3 MIN) PAGE 176

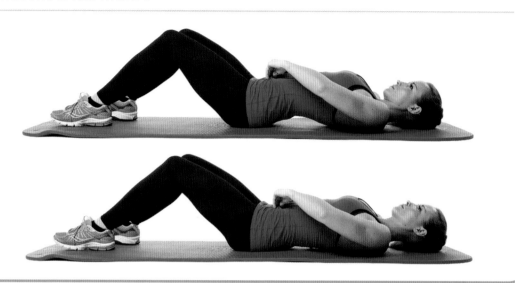

17. Hamstring/core combination
(STRENGTH) (1.5 MIN) PAGE 177

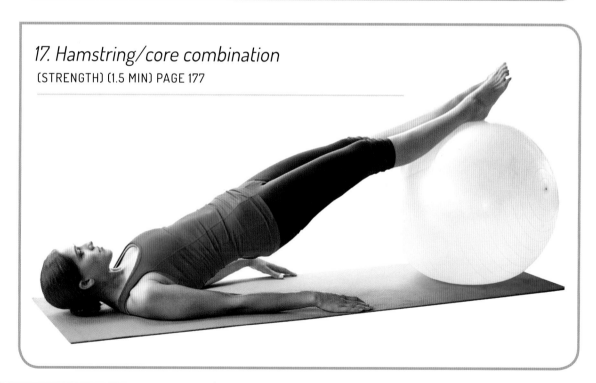

18. Glutes
(STRETCH) (30 SEC X 3 OR 45 SEC X 2) PAGE 177

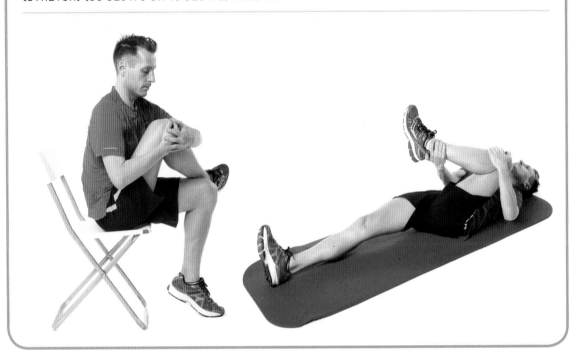

19. Hamstring
(STRETCH) (1.5 MIN) PAGE 178

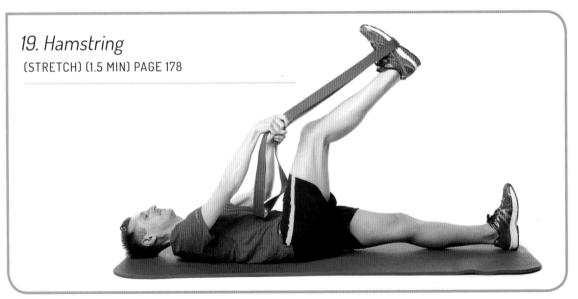

20. ITB Tensor Fascia Latae (TFL)
(STRETCH) (30 SEC X 3) PAGE 178

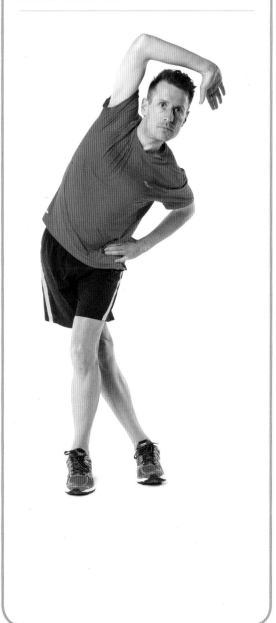

21. Side step with squat
(STRENGTH) (4 MIN) PAGE 179

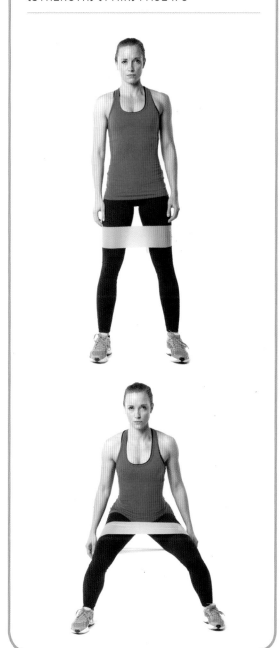

VISITING THE PHYSIOTHERAPIST: GOOD PRACTICE

This is to assist you if you haven't ever been to see a physiotherapist before. Its intention is to expedite the process for you so you get the maximum benefit from your visit.

1) Consider what injury it is that you want to speak to the physiotherapist about. This may seem simple, but believe it or not, it is quite rare to have a new client attend and present just one injury. A physiotherapist faced with one main issue is targeted and time rich, whereas when we are overloaded with a series of unrelated injuries, the appointment time appears to shrink and the key reason for your visit can be lost in the explanation.

   This is not to say that pain felt elsewhere other than your key injury site is not relevant, but be clear from the outset what your main focus for the visit is.

2) Read up a little before arrival. It can be very helpful to have a patient who has a greater understanding of his or her symptoms and can allow us to dispel some myths from Google at the outset, or to confirm their suspicions and self-diagnosis as true.

3) Be a good historian. Thinking ahead of the visit about when your pain first came on, any potential contributing causes you can think of; and bringing any paperwork you have such as scan results or medication lists is always very helpful.

4) Choose your clothes wisely. Physiotherapists are very used to moving patients' clothing appropriately to work on clients, however, for you it may well be a new experience. In most cases, I will want to look at the skin. This means at the very least lifting a garment out of the way, so if you have a knee problem, taking shorts to change into is a great idea, or a vest top for women with a shoulder issue. There are always those who don't care, for example, many triathletes are often stripping off before we have finished talking about the injury! It is our job as physio to reboot each time and be respectful of your choices, so please put everyone at ease and think about this beforehand, putting yourself fully in control of the situation.

5) Make notes when you are with us, this allows you to ask all questions throughout your treatment process and of course remember what you have heard when you get home. Confirm and paraphrase what you think you are supposed to be doing between sessions, this way everyone knows what is expected and how we intend to proceed.

6) Ask how many sessions we think it will take, it's OK to provide rough parameters based upon experience of the same condition. You may of course be cured early or perhaps have to stay on for one or two additional sessions.

RUNNING FREE OF INJURIES

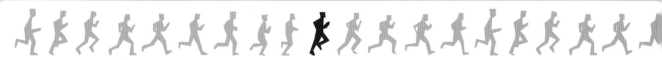

With these helpful tips, everyone will get the most out of the experience and you should get the best value for your money.

The following is a helpful guide to the way a physiotherapist will interact with you, so you are prepared for the jargon.

We work out how bad an injury is on the basis of severity, irritability and the nature of the pain (S.I.N.). Whilst we need you to be a good historian regarding your injury, we also want to question you as to how bad it feels and when you do something that aggravates it, how long that takes and then how long before it settles down. If we can assess how painful it is, what makes it worse and how quickly it settles, it enables us to start formulating a plan for the treatment. The nature of the pain depends upon where we feel the pain is being generated. You feel pain in different ways and will describe it differently. The words you use to describe your pain make all the difference to us, from stabbing, electric, burning pain to a dull ache. We rate pain from 0–10, zero being no pain at all and ten being the most pain you can imagine. This is called the visual analogue scale (VAS) for pain (Hawker *et al.*, 2011).

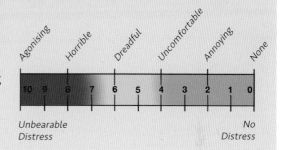

Coping with Injury

When you get injured it is important to stay connected to the sport you love. Always continue to stay involved with your running club, whether it's helping out with the warm-up exercises or doing some timing for the group. Staying connected to the group is shown to reduce the depressed feelings you have when injured and keeps you motivated to return to the sport as soon as possible.

Be realistic about the injury. If a trained professional is telling you that it will take six weeks then do not fall into the trap of believing that you are going to do it in five in some sort of competition that this will make you seem better than all others. The likely outcome is that you will reinjure yourself and face another six weeks sidelined for the sake of one week more rehabilitation. Instead, map out your programme for the six weeks that will enable you return to your usual programme. Write it up and tick off the mini goals that you achieve along the way. For example, ticking off doing your home exercise programme daily – whilst a small goal – is a very pragmatic step to becoming injury-free. Cross training keeps you connected to your fitness goals, so swim, row, aqua jog your way to improved fitness until you are ready to run again.

Being injured can be a difficult time, and people can become tetchy and irritable and difficult to be around, often taking out their frustrations on others. This is not inevitable. Choose to be upbeat, pragmatic and focused on getting back to full health, keep the glass half full and find as many ways as possible to fill it up again rather than becoming yet another moody injured runner. We learn far more about our abilities when we are down than when we are setting a new personal best.

So, let's get started, with each common running injury from the foot up.

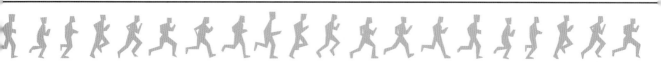

CHAPTER 1

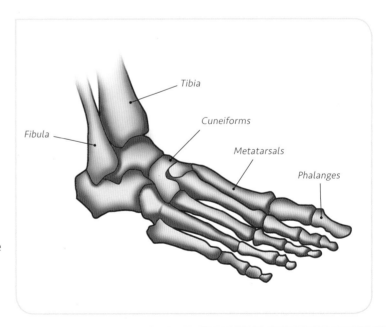

THE FOOT

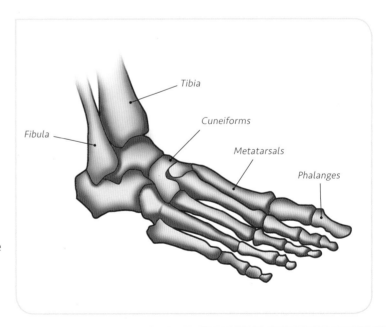

The foot. What a structure! This is the foundation of your body, the bedrock of your running movement and arguably the most expensive part of the body given the cost of running shoes these days. The thing about the foot is that we are capable of ignoring aches and pains around it due to that fact we spend so much time standing. It can appear quite normal for a foot to ache at the end of a long day at work or after exercising, and kicking off your shoes and just having a good rub can work wonders. But what happens when something else is going on? How do we differentiate a mild ache from something that is likely to stop us running for a while?

The issues that affect the foot are plentiful. Here are the most common injuries of the foot (not in order of prevalence) that affect the keen runner:

- Morton's neuroma
- Plantar fasciitis
- Hallux valgus/bunions (with note to Hallux rigidus)
- Metatarsal stress fracture
- Cuboid syndrome.

Barefoot Running and Minimalist Footwear

Before we get onto each of these injuries, there is a great deal of discussion surrounding footwear, – conventional, minimalist footwear and barefoot running. Be aware that barefoot running and minimalist footwear are not the same; when I refer

Tibia

Cuneiforms

Fibula

Metatarsals

Phalanges

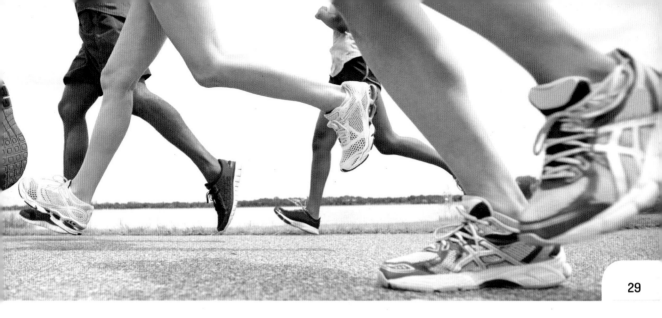

to barefoot running I am talking about running with nothing at all on the foot.

Let's tackle barefoot running first. We all like something that is new and sensational and there are a select group of people who will always want to be ground breakers.

Barefoot running has been shown to reduce forces through the knee, but appears to increase forces and tension within the foot and Achilles tendon (Kulmala *et al.*, 2013). It is my contention that barefoot running is a training aid. It doesn't make you injury-free. Pro-barefoot runners make much of strengthening exercises, but for a committed runner that strengthening should be done anyway.

For those who want to move to barefoot running, it has to be done properly, with personalized advice, attention to your biomechanics and appropriate strength and conditioning training before and during the transition. We modern-day consumers like convenience and speed in everything we do. I believe that barefoot running should be seen as a training aid to strengthen the foot as part of a good strength and conditioning programme, or left to those who have been habitual barefoot runners/walkers from birth (Leiberman *et al.*, 2010). We can't be lazy when it comes to rehab and strength and conditioning (S&C) exercises; they take time out of

our day to do properly and should be additional to our running plan. What takes a great deal more time – six to nine months – is to properly make a change from using a shoe to running in a minimalist sock or totally barefoot. On that basis, I just don't see it being successful or popular for long.

If you don't agree, just look at the start of any elite race across the globe, you will not see a single top-flight athlete running barefoot. With their scientific support and multimillion-pound contracts, elite athletes are all focused on two things: success and career longevity. Therefore nobody can have offered them sufficient proof that barefoot running will achieve faster times or reduce injury. Nobody has convinced me either.

Barefoot is different to minimalist footwear. Minimalist footwear relates to shoes with minimal support or cushioning. These are commonplace in elite start lines and are favoured as they are light, provide freedom of movement and do not hinder natural running technique. In fact, there is evidence to back this lack of support. There is some benefit to biomechanics, speed and running efficiency. Most of the research has looked at ground reaction forces, concluding in many cases that a change in footwear to a more minimalist approach doesn't affect the way you strike your foot, though some argue there is a reduction in cushioning (O'Leary *et al.*, 2008). It

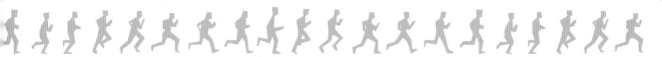

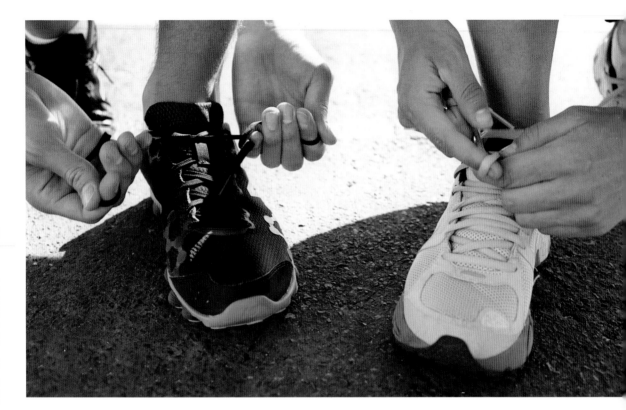

is the likely technical improvements that come with the change (Myer *et al.*, 2012), causing the reduction in ground reaction forces that potentially reduce injury. Strengthening your body and improving technique will help you more than changing your shoes; but a structured approach to both may have the greatest benefit of all. Just as you should save before you buy something, rather than go into debt, you must train to be a better runner. Spending money on shoes and expecting them to make you faster is not the answer. As research develops we will understand more about this en vogue topic, however I suspect more minimalist footwear will become the norm, barefoot running will only be used as a training aid, and runners will eventually abandon motion control footwear and heavy, clumpy support shoes.

The barefoot lobby base their advocacy partly on the notion that Kenyans (amongst runners of other African nations) run barefoot and that's why they are the best runners in the world, coupled with the potential reduction in ground reaction forces and resultant reduced injury potential (Czyzewski, 2012).

However, Kenyan runners also eat large volumes of ugali (a high-carbohydrate, rich food), walk on softer, more natural surfaces than concrete, and many live at altitude, running more as a consequence of their daily routine than as a stress release at the end of the day. One of the most significant sporting opportunities available to an athletic Kenyan is to become an elite runner. This opportunity helps to focus the talent of the nation so that the very best runners come to the front, not just the ones who didn't make it as a football player or rugby star.

As such, I don't think that the sole reason that Kenyans are brilliant runners is because they run barefoot, particularly when, as soon as they can get their hands on trainers, they wear them. Other runners, such as Olympic and World Champion Mo Farah, habitually wear shoes and trainers and he has beaten them at their own game.

It's hugely interesting that one nation has such a high proportion of the best long distance runners in the world and hopefully more research is undertaken to find out why. We study these athletes and their feet, assuming they have a certain foot type because they are Kenyan or that their biomechanics are so good because of their childhood, but what if we studied the very best European and American athletes and included the very top of the tree in all sports? What would we find from looking at Ronaldo, Wilkinson, the Brownlee brothers, Djokovic, the winner of the Marathon de Sables, Olympic medalists in badminton, even Bradley Wiggins and other non-running athletes? It is possible that if all this talent were to be channeled into the sport of running instead of thinly spread across many, there would be faster times and less dominance from some of the African nations. Without the lure of so many other sports to tempt individuals away from the lesser paid sport of running, how well would Europeans and Americans actually perform?

So as I step down from my soapbox, let's get back to the foot and running-related injuries.

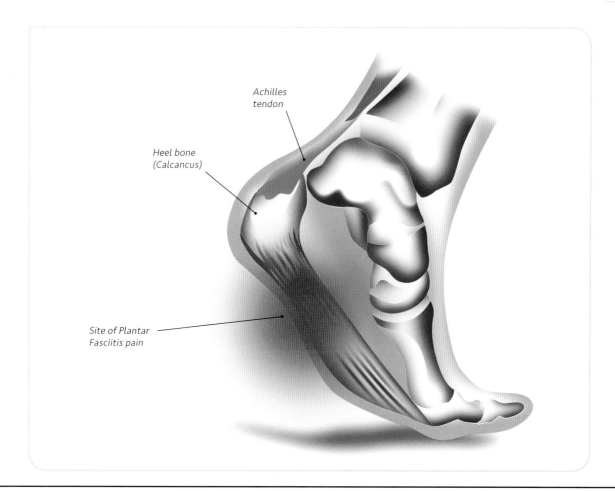

Achilles tendon

Heel bone (Calcancus)

Site of Plantar Fasciitis pain

Morton's Neuroma

What is it?

A neuroma is an abnormal enlargement of nerve tissue. Nerves are the motor and sensory carrying structures of the body. This means that in order for us to move, or feel, we need nerves to send the messages with the relevant information to the required muscle groups. This information to and from the brain provides immediate information back and forth to create and moderate movement, touch, temperature, proprioception (where your limb is in space) and sensation.

A Morton's neuroma can be described as a thickening or swelling of the tiny little nerve that passes between your toe joints. Usually it's between the third and fourth metatarsals but can also be between the second and third metatarsals. (The big toe is always number one, the little toe number five – the same with the thumb, one, and little finger, five, in the hand.) The pain radiates along the two affected toes and is sore on the underside of the foot at the location of the neuroma.

When a nerve develops a neuroma there is greater surface area of the nerve, an increased likelihood of entrapment and constant pressure, which reduces the ability of the nerve to slide efficiently between neighbouring structures.

It's not overly common as an injury in clinic, but there are significant numbers of people who present with foot pain in this area, so let's discuss the signs and symptoms so you don't overlook this possible diagnosis.

EARLY WARNING SIGNS

- Pain between the metatarsal heads of toes two three or three–four
- Numbness in the area
- Feeling that something is in your shoe under the ball of the foot
- Tingling or pins and needles in the toes.

COMMON REASONS FOR INJURY

- Wearing tight or pointed footwear
- High heel shoes
- Repetitive movements such as running or racquet sports

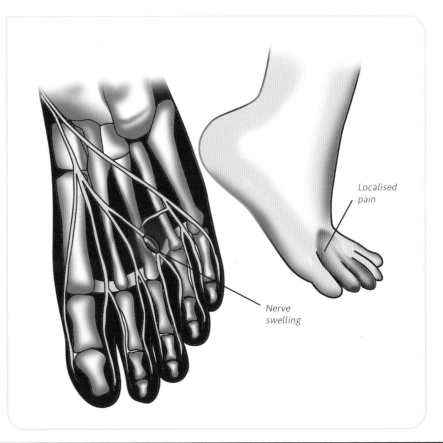

Localised pain

Nerve swelling

- Injury or trauma to the foot
- Foot abnormalities such as bunions, flat foot or over-flexible feet.

It should be noted that not all pain in the toes can be linked to a neuroma, however, as a runner this would be one to watch out for.

Of course not all forefoot pain is due to a neuroma, but there can be an audible click when the toes are squeezed that is a good clinical way of determining if further investigation is warranted along with the clinical presentation (a clinical presentation is largely information gained from the client describing what's wrong, and the therapist drawing parallels with each potential diagnosis, then testing structures to narrow that diagnosis). The audible click in the metatarsal heads when we squeeze the toes would lead a physio to perform an ultrasound scan. The ultrasound scan is a method of looking beneath the skin into the structures of the foot, the same as scans done during pregnancy to look at a baby. The ultrasound can show the structures moving and, in the case of a Morton's neuroma when performing the squeeze test, show the neuroma try to move between the metatarsal bones, confirming our diagnosis.

PROGRESSION OF THE INJURY

The injury starts very slowly, and often just removing your shoes and rubbing your foot is enough to alleviate the symptoms in the early days. There may be significant breaks in the symptoms so you may at first believe that it's just a problem with a certain pair of shoes. The symptoms will then worsen over time and become more consistent. The temporary changes to the nerve will begin to become more permanent and your pain will become more constant. All movement can become painful and you will avoid putting any pressure on your forefoot.

SELF-ASSESSMENT

Take your foot into your hand and squeeze the toes together. If you feel or hear a click as you squeeze, then you may have this condition. Seek medical advice from a physiotherapist.

TREATMENT

As with all injuries, early detection is very important. The sooner a specialist can diagnose Morton's neuroma, the better chance you have of reducing the need for surgery.

Treatment is not normally through physiotherapy. Initially orthotics (insoles) can be used to hold your foot in a specific position in order to open the toes so the nerve is no longer being squashed. Another common method of treatment is to inject the neuroma, either with a steroid to reduce the inflammation or with a 4% ethyl alcohol solution to 'deaden' the nerve and therefore reduce the pain sensation.

If these fail, then an operation is used to excise the unwanted material, however, in some cases the scar tissue from the operation can cause as many issues as the neuroma did beforehand, which is why it is so important to rest post-operatively and to perform specific exercises to mobilize the soft tissues. With surgery there is the option of going in via the top (dorsum) of the foot and sacrificing a ligament that stops your toes from splaying, (though subsequent shoe compression will reduce this issue), or the underside (plantar) of the foot (Wu, 2009); however, this takes longer to heal after surgery. Personally, I would inject and use orthotics together to try and solve this issue, stop the sufferer wearing tight-fitting shoes and trust that the injections reduce the size of the neuroma or surrounding tissues.

SELF-TREATMENT

There is very little that you can do, besides wearing wide, cushioned footwear and moderating your activity until you see a professional. If you suspect a Morton's neuroma, stop running so that you reduce the irritation and make an appointment to see a physiotherapist as soon as possible. Avoid high heel shoes and tight-fitting shoes until the diagnosis has been confirmed.

Exercises to assist with associated musculoskeletal disorders as a result of having a Morton's neuroma would be: Towel grabbing (strength), p. 167, Calf (stretch) p. 168, Soleus

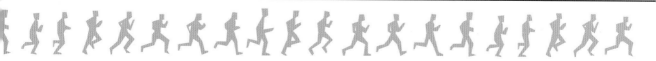

(stretch), p. 168, The clam – hip abduction/rotation (strength), p. 173, Core muscles (strength), p. 176.

WHAT TO EXPECT FROM A PHYSIOTHERAPIST

This is largely going to be assessment and – in the absence of your physio having an ultrasound-scanning device – onward referral. There is the opportunity to have some soft tissue work (specific massage to the area) on the lower leg, reducing tension in the muscles to prevent associated injury from you mechanically offloading your foot with a different walking posture. I always suggest calf stretches for the reduction in forefoot load. Physiotherapists and podiatrists would look closely at the reasons for this occurrence, assess your footwear and the ankle, knee and hip joints to look for clues as to why this might have occurred.

Therapy can be therefore be directed at the cause in order to prevent it happening again, offering you some concurrent rehabilitation alongside the treatment to the small neuroma in the foot.

GETTING BACK TO RUNNING

The length of time it will take to get back to running? As with many injuries, how long is a

PRACTITIONER PROTOCOL

In this instance, the diagnosis is the best opportunity for you to be effective along with footwear advice.

- Refer for an ultrasound scan to confirm diagnosis
- Give advice on shoes with a more open toe box and cushioning
- Refer for podiatry assessment
- Explain the options:
  — Injection
  — Surgery
  — Conservative approach
- Suggest additional help in the form of:
  — Soft tissue release
  — Foot and ankle mobilization
  — Moderation of activity.

In the event that the person affected would like some supporting treatments I suggest the following:

- Soft tissue massage to the gastrocnemius and soleus
- Frictions to the dorsal tendons and release of anterior muscles
- Gentle massage of the plantar fascia
- Talocrural and sub talar mobilization
- Tarsal joint global mobilization.

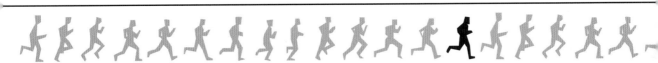

I have been fit and active all my life enjoying a variety of sports including walking, cycling and classes at the local gym. A lot of my work has also been on my feet. In my early fifties I began to feel discomfort in the ball of my right foot.

Over several months the discomfort increased, feeling like I had a small pebble in my shoe. I allowed months to pass, continuing to exercise, but the problem became worse. I tried different trainers and different insoles in my shoes. I saw a podiatrist and had special insoles made but none of this really helped the pain, which came with any pressure on the foot. I began to experience excruciating pains as soon as my foot touched the ground and even sometimes at rest.

I mentioned my problems to an instructor at a class and he recommended Paul as he had seen him regarding his own musculoskeletal problems. When I saw him, Paul listened carefully to my list of aches and pains. On examination, when my toes were squeezed there was an audible click. Paul suspected

a Morton's neuroma and suggested an ultrasound scan to investigate further. He also worked on my foot and in further sessions helped my knees and hips as well as giving me exercises to follow at home. The scan confirmed the Morton's neuroma and a cortisone injection was suggested. The first one had minimal effect and the second one caused fat wasting and further pain.

After further sessions with Paul, he suggested seeing an orthopaedic surgeon. In the end, I had surgery to remove the neuroma, after which the pain was much decreased, especially the sharp nerve pain, though I am still left with some numbness around the area and discomfort on the ball of my foot. I continue to wear orthotic insoles to accommodate the shape of my foot, which helps and has allowed me to take up most of my previous activities.

I am now aware that I have extremely mobile joints in my feet and the excessive movement coupled with the lack of padding has contributed to my developing this problem.

piece of string? But usually six weeks post-surgery will see a return to the cross trainer. Some people, however, have suffered swelling and soreness up to a year post-surgery. I would conservatively estimate that 12 weeks post-surgery you could expect to be back running, sooner if there are no complications.

Plantar fasciitis

What is it?

Plantar fasciitis is an injury to the thick fascia band that passes from the heel bone to the toes along the bottom (plantar) of your foot. It has a couple of key roles, firstly to protect the foot, but also to maintain the tension in the longitudinal arch of the foot. It

assists with the propulsive forces of the foot during walking or running.

Plantar fasciitis is inflammation and damage to the connective tissue known as the plantar fascia. There is some fairly new information emerging that suggests the damage to the plantar fascia comes about through degeneration of the fascia rather than a traumatic event. Running is one of the greatest risk factors, along with standing for long periods, and it's often known as 'jogger's heel' or 'policeman's heel' for these reasons.

EARLY WARNING SIGNS

- A sharp pain on the inside of the heel just as the longitudinal arch starts
- Feeling of standing on a stone in the morning
- Pain wears off after a few steps and seems to be fine for the rest of the day

- First step pain can occur after any reasonable length of rest.

COMMON REASONS FOR INJURY

The biggest risk factor for plantar fasciitis has been shown to be a loss of dorsiflexion. Dorsiflexion is the ankle movement upward toward the shin, resulting in a stretch to the posterior structures in the lower leg, namely the calf muscles. The second greatest risk factor for plantar fasciitis is a higher body mass index (BMI) (Riddle *et al.*, 2003).

There is also a strong association with people who have flatter feet (Warren, 1990), which is a lack of height within the longitudinal arch of the foot, or who have excessively high arches.

This places more stress on the plantar fascia and therefore the damage or degeneration occurs. With runners, or those who are overweight, the pressure is built up due to additional strain on the fascia as the foot tries to accept the increased load. So if you are carrying a bit of extra weight, have taken up running and have flat feet, beware the early morning feeling of standing on a stone.

PROGRESSION OF THE INJURY

- The pain ceases to wear off after a few steps in the morning and can continue well into your day.
- After a while this pain becomes more consistent and even hurts after a short period of sitting or driving.
- The pain is unremitting and prevents you from walking any distance at all, with the sufferer even resorting to crutches in the most severe of cases.

SELF-ASSESSMENT

Imagine your heel pad as a clock face, with the Achilles at 6 o'clock. Place your fingers over 1 o'clock on the left foot or 10 o'clock on the right foot and press in this location. If you have immediate

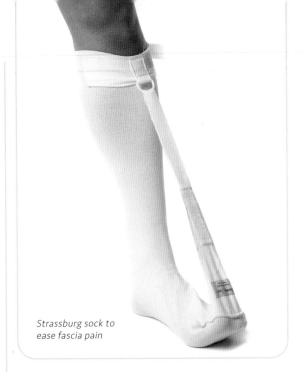

Strassburg sock to ease fascia pain

pain, there is a high chance you have plantar fasciitis as this is the typical location of pain for the majority of sufferers.

With your foot placed on the floor, pull up your big toe. If you feel pain in this same location, then this is further evidence to support the diagnosis. If you have pain in this area during the first few steps in the morning, I would consider this as plantar fasciitis.

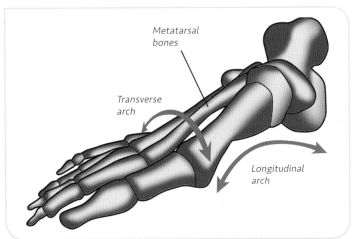

Metatarsal bones

Transverse arch

Longitudinal arch

TREATMENT

Treatment for plantar fasciitis is one of those where health care professionals vary dramatically in their thinking. I once had a heated debate with someone who I admire greatly owing to my claims that I could successfully treat plantar fasciitis. I was speaking as a physio, using my own protocol derived from literature and experience, while he, a podiatrist with an amazing reputation, was talking about his specialist area of the foot.

The first time I had someone come in to my clinic with plantar fasciitis I didn't do anything for them, and as a consequence never saw them again. In my defence, the received wisdom back in those days was to do nothing, as, after all, this is a self-limiting condition, so I had explained to this client that in eighteen months to three years it would disappear of its own volition and until then he shouldn't run. His reply has never left me; he told me that, as a runner, that line of attack wasn't an option and that he would have to do something, anything!

I set about reading everything I could on the subject. There were clearly therapists trying different approaches, but the recurrent theme was 'no running'. My searches led me to the *Runner's World* online forum on plantar fasciitis, where there were literally tens of thousands of entries on this subject alone. Many runners had also been told to stop running by health care practitioners. I was horrified at the volume of people suffering and at the end of their tether following months and even years of fruitless searching for something more pragmatic than rest.

I therefore developed a protocol for plantar fasciitis that I have modified over the last 10 years. Because this protocol is something I have put together myself, I have to spell this out to patients who attend my clinic so they understand that it hasn't been tested or peer-reviewed like other treatments on offer.

I can't cure plantar fasciitis but I have had a great deal of success with a large number of clients who followed this protocol. It won't differ greatly from what everyone else is doing these days, but I maintain that 10 years ago, a lot of physiotherapy departments were opting for the 'wait and see' approach and it was the podiatry clinics that were leading the way. I learned a great deal from research produced from foot and ankle specialists and used their knowledge to produce changes to this protocol.

SHOCKWAVE THERAPY

There is a growing body of evidence to show that extracorporeal shockwave therapy (ECSWT – or SWT for short) is an excellent treatment for plantar fasciitis. I have been so gripped by the ability of this treatment that mine was one of the first physiotherapy clinics in the UK to buy a machine and my results (anecdotally) have been nothing short of incredible, not just with plantar fasciitis but with a wide range of soft tissue and bone injuries.

Shockwave therapy has until recently had some pretty sketchy results from the scientific world. Recent studies performed to a high standard have resulted in the National Institute for Care and Excellence (N.I.C.E.) guidelines being updated. Some of their published studies are citing 75-85% of patients pain-free on six-month follow-up after shockwave therapy treatments. I was so encouraged by these statistics that I invested in a Shockwave machine myself for my clinic. I am getting much higher percentages of improvement, with significantly faster results than the studies show, and I believe this will be the treatment of choice for those whose plantar fasciitis fails to respond to the usual treatments. Shockwave therapy should not be used within twelve weeks of an injection to the area so it is also my treatment choice ahead of injection, which has only limited support from the scientific community.

How SWT works is not 100% known, however, it is believed that it stimulates the immune system and releases nucleic acids within the target cells, which in non-scientific terms are the prerequisites for any tissue healing. In order for healing to take place this process must occur and with SWT the initial process is one of mechanical pressure, which increases the cell permeability, increasing local circulation to the tissues and increasing metabolism.

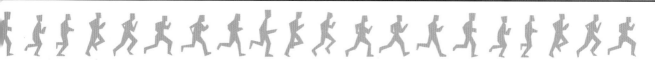

Second, it breaks up any calcium deposits through the pressure, producing hundreds of thousands of cavitational bubbles that expand and then collapse creating a secondary force breaking up the calcific deposits. Cells responsible for soft tissue and bone regeneration and healing are known as fibroblasts and osteoblasts. SWT has been shown to stimulate these cells and therefore promote healing on a grand scale. Finally, SWT has a pain-reducing element to it, working on the brain's transmission of pain; first of all as a transient, short-lived pain reduction, but it has also been shown to work on the 'pain-gate', acting as a reset button for the perception of pain and therefore having potential long-term effects on pain reduction.

SELF-TREATMENT

Plantar fasciitis protocol – the 10-point plan:

1   No barefoot walking, not ever, not even for a midnight trip to the bathroom
2   Wear orthotic insoles (off the shelf Scholl orthoheels are fine initially) in all your shoes to support the foot's arch

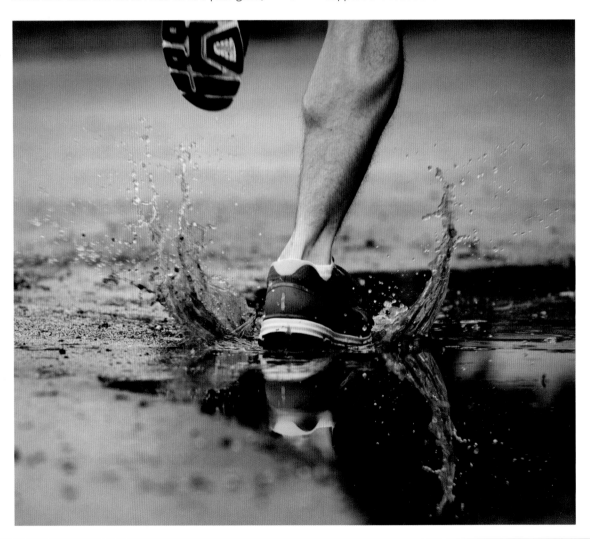

3   Before moving after a period of rest, write the alphabet with your foot in mid air
4   Stretch your calf 6 times per day for 45 seconds. See page 168
5   Soleus stretch 6 times per day for 45 seconds. See page 168
6   Drag a towel along the floor with your toes for 2 minutes twice a day. See page 167
7   Ice the foot after any significant period of standing or walking
8   Have weekly treatments involving:
    a) Soft tissue massage to the gastrocnemius and soleus
    b) Soft tissue massage to the underside of the foot (the plantar) but not the immediate area of pain
    c) Transverse frictions over the site of pain for up to 2 minutes until numbing is achieved (the pain has gone; if the physio has slipped off the area of pain, tell them) then 10 minutes of frictions (if chronic)
9   Wear a Strassburg Sock (see page 36) at night to keep a mild stretch on the fascia overnight
10 Use anti-inflammatory medication if you can without side-effects, as directed by your GP.

The aim of the protocol is to:

- increase range of movement in the soft tissues to reduce the stress placed at the site of injury
- encourage healing at a cellular level, developing the collagen fibres that make up the fascia
- support the longitudinal arch of the foot and reduce the strain being placed at the site of injury, and to lengthen and strengthen the soft tissues providing a mechanically robust foot and ankle.

The pre-movement warming up increases blood flow and makes tissue more pliable and less likely to rupture, just like when you warm up prior to a run.

This fairly obvious and intuitive approach lacks the introduction of running to the programme.

Where podiatrists and I agree is that you need to take an initial rest from running which can be very demoralizing for runners. Repair cannot be attained at any level if excessive forces are being placed through the plantar fasciitis on a regular basis. There are greater than double the forces placed through the PF when running compared to walking. However, there does come a time when I will start the patient back on the road. Though some practitioners will leave the running until you can push the injured area and feel nothing, I will allow some rehabilitation runs to take place once you are walking pain-free and don't have the morning 'standing on a stone' pain any more.

WHAT TO EXPECT FROM A PHYSIOTHERAPIST

There are some pretty basic tests to assess for plantar fasciitis, and the client's story usually confirms the diagnosis quite easily, but an ultrasound scan is what truly confirms the extent of the injury. Treatment in my clinic is weekly as outlined in the protocol and all the exercises and treatments are outlined here.

GETTING BACK TO RUNNING

The gradual return to running is based upon two key parameters; starting early enough to maintain the muscle strength and conditioning that has been built through pre-injury running, whilst not overloading the fascia so as to cause too much trauma and thus prolonging the period of injury.

When you are running regularly, you condition your body through event-specific strength and local muscular endurance. Rest brings with it a detraining effect no matter how diligent you are at doing a home-based exercise programme (HEP). It is my contention that by stopping someone from running altogether for a long period, you in fact exacerbate this detraining effect and the potential weakness that may have facilitated the injury in the first place is now worse than before. Of course we can work really hard to maintain core strength, leg strength and the like, using a robust set of assessment techniques to identify any such weakness. Biomechanical irregularities can be assessed and we work hard to ensure that the individual returns to their pre-injured condition in a better state than before. However,

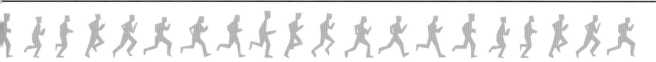

PRACTITIONER PROTOCOL

Use my 10-point plan initially:

1) No barefoot walking
2) Wear orthotic insoles
3) Warm up with writing alphabet with foot after any period of rest
4) Stretch Gastrocnemius 6 times per day – Calf (stretch), page 168
5) Stretch your soleus 6 times per day – Soleus (stretch), page 168
6) Towel grabbing for 2 minutes twice a day, page 167
7) Ice the foot after any significant period of standing or walking for 12 minutes
8) Treatments weekly for 5–15 weeks.

The treatments should include:

a. Specific Soft Tissue Massage to the gastrocnemius and soleus (SSTM)
b. SSTM to the underside of the plantar avoiding the origin
c. Deep Transverse Frictions (DTF) to the origin if chronic.

I recommend 3 shockwave therapy sessions of 500 shocks at 1.5htz and then 2000 shocks at 2.5htz.

9) Wear a Strassburg Sock at night (see page 46)
10) Use anti-inflammatory medication as directed by your GP.

as good as we all are, can such efforts be any real substitute for the benefits of running?

The development of the anti-gravity treadmills and aqua jogging belts would suggest that science supports using the most specific form of training at your disposal. The cost of anti-gravity treadmills (where you run whilst partially suspended) makes them a professional athletes' choice, so what can we lesser mortals do instead?

Rehab runs, that are short in duration, offer regular stops for stretching and pain recording. The idea is that if you notice an increase in pain levels, then you either stop, see if stretching benefits your foot, or within certain parameters continue for another rep.

Recommended running programme: 3 minutes steady jog. Stretch gastrocnemius and soleus, 30 seconds each x 2 as described in the exercise appendix – Calf (stretch), page 168, Soleus (stretch), page 168.

In order to understand when you have to stop, use a pain rating system that physiotherapists call the visual analogue scale for pain (VAS). The scale is 0 through to 10, zero being no pain at all and 10 being the most pain you can imagine. '3/10 VAS' indicates a score of 3 out of 10.

You can repeat this self-assessment run up to a maximum of five times. If the discomfort comes on immediately, then you must stop. If there is a gradual ache that doesn't rise above 3/10 on the

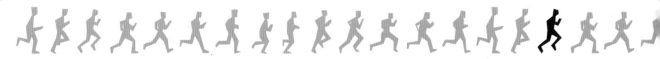

visual analogue scale, then you can continue as long as the pain doesn't build from there. If the pain is rising all the time, despite the stretch stops, even if it doesn't rise above the 3/10 VAS, then you should stop.

These runs can be repeated after two full days of rest. Typically, you will not manage all five runs for at least two weeks. Once all five runs have been completed within the parameters, you can increase the running time to 4 minutes, then 5 minutes and so on, reducing the sets as you progress, so the total time doesn't become unmanageable. Once you have reached 4 x 10 minutes, move to 2 x 20 minutes, then 1 x 30 minutes, 3 x 20 minutes, etc.

This process, can sometimes feel like one step forwards, two steps back. I believe that if you rest without running at all and wait for the pain to have totally gone, you will lose a lot of the lower leg strength you've gained, which is a key component for good running biomechanics. My argument is that without any running as part of your rehabilitation, the fascia hasn't had to respond to any stress akin to running for such a long time that this increases the risk of re-injury. There are risks associated with my protocol; however, the injury risk is mitigated by slowly loading the PF with short bouts of jogging and by keeping the soft tissues long by regular intervals of stretching. From my experience with patients, the double rest days allow repair to any new micro-trauma and ensure the process is fairly robust.

Starting to run whilst there is still a small amount of pain is often rejected as an option by therapists as they do not wish to take the risk, so you have two options immediately open to you:

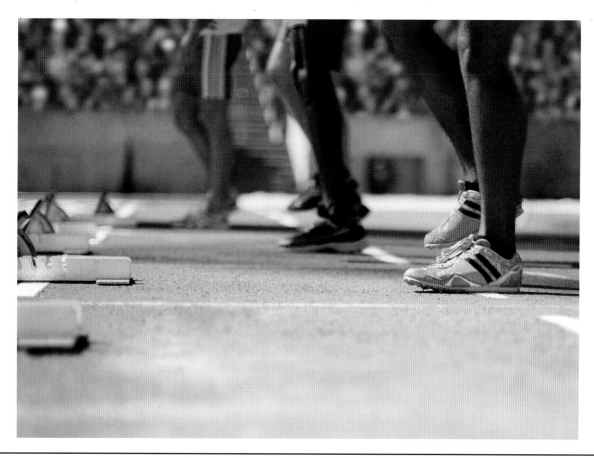

1. Rest until you have been pain-free for two weeks and then start back gradually
2. Use my option of gradually returning to running once you reach the milestone of pain-free walking and manageable pain levels during running. This is only whilst under strict supervision and being 100% committed to the regime outlined later in this section.

Option three is to look at steroid injections or shockwave therapy; in short, throw the kitchen sink at the issue (and some money) if conservative physiotherapy fails.

CLIENT STORY: SARITA, 37

When I was 33 and after 10 years of trying through the ballot, I got a place in the 2011 London Marathon. A regular runner, I went from running twice a week to training four times a week.

I felt some niggling pain in my foot, but I ignored it because over the years I had on occasion felt a twinge, but it had always gone away straight away. Sometimes it was OK to run on, and sometimes it would cause me to stop running and walk for a bit, but then be able to run again.

In the end my training became severely affected. I was in agony not only when I was running but also in everyday life. From the moment I woke up I was getting sharp pain, pulling pain and just outright agony in my foot. It was so bad at times that I ended up limping, not wearing shoes or having only to wear trainers with a little more arch support. None of which really seemed to ease it. I tried painkillers at times because it was so bad, but they didn't really help it.

I went to a sports shop to get myself some new trainers, thinking that might be the issue and told them about the pain I was getting. Luckily, Physio&Therapy UK were operating from the back of the shop. The physio diagnosed it as plantar fasciitis and said I would need treatment.

As the weeks went on things didn't improve so I made an appointment to see the physio. I had a few sessions, at which the physio massaged my calf and foot, which can only be described as excruciating,

and some regular exercises to do every day, twice a day. And he also gave me a rather 'attractive' sock to wear at night to stretch out my muscle. He also explained exactly what had happened to my foot, and what it would look like inside, which I found really useful and interesting.

I had to, under advice, give up running for about four to six weeks, which was a nightmare whilst training for a marathon. All I could do was cross train in the gym. I was getting really anxious about the race, as it had been a lifelong ambition for me, but I kept up with the exercises and the sock and got myself to the start line.

I'm not going to say that on race day my foot didn't hurt because it did, but it wasn't nearly as bad as it had been. I probably shouldn't have run but I was never not going to. I got round, and finished the race – which to this date is the best feeling I've ever had. I wasn't quick, and I did walk in places, and I did stop to stretch my foot with the exercises I had been shown on a couple of occasions, but I did it.

I then took a couple of weeks off running and, apart from a couple of twinges, I haven't had any further pain since. I train three times a week, stretching my foot with the same exercises I was shown before each run. And I've completed several half marathons (my half marathon PB is 2.07), lots of 10 mile and 5k races, all without pain!

Hallux valgus/bunions and hallux rigidus

What is it?

Hallux valgus is the condition where the first metatarsal deviates towards the other foot, the big toe moves the other way towards the toes and the joint becomes prominent on the inside. Whilst there can be some bone growth, it is effectively the joint being out of position that causes the lump.

Hallux limitus/rigidus, is, as the name suggests, a rigidity of the big toe. Consider the main phases of walking and you will see the relevance that a loss of movement in this joint has to you as a runner.

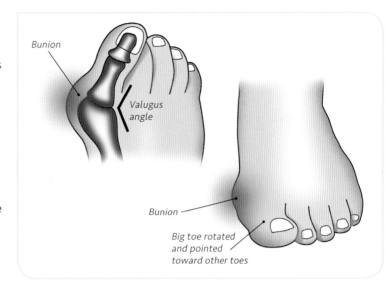

Bunion

Valugus angle

Bunion

Big toe rotated and pointed toward other toes

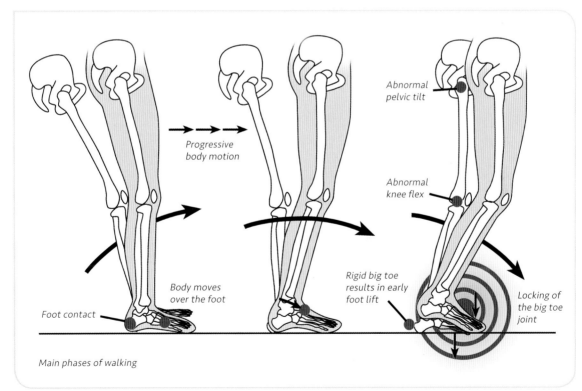

Progressive body motion

Abnormal pelvic tilt

Abnormal knee flex

Body moves over the foot

Foot contact

Rigid big toe results in early foot lift

Locking of the big toe joint

Main phases of walking

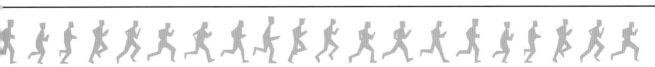

EARLY WARNING SIGNS/ RISK FACTORS OF HALLUX VALGUS

It is very difficult to notice the mild changes in a big toe over time. It's probably better to look at your risk factors associated with the issue.

- Do you wear high heels, pointed or tight fitting shoes?
- Do your parents or older siblings have this issue?
- Do both of your feet look identical; is one big toe slightly more laterally rotated than the other?

You will be at a higher risk if you can answer yes to two out of three of these questions. In the majority of cases, the person reading this will already know they have a bunion or a slightly abducted big toe.

One of the best methods of assessing this issue is to keep checking your feet, look for abnormalities and changes over time. Pain or blisters can add to this clinical history and help build a picture of future issues.

Hallux rigidus will cause issues through the running gait, with early warning signs of:

- Tension in the calf
- Plantar fascia pain
- Overload of the knee causing pain
- Potentially lower back pain.

COMMON REASONS FOR INJURY FROM HALLUX VALGUS

Most people agree that there is a hereditary aspect to this (Piqué-Vidal *et al.*, 2007), but interestingly a study back in 1952 found that for West Africans who did not wear shoes, the valgus angles of the big toe (inward movement as shown above) were not present in any age or gender. In cultures where shoes are commonplace from a young age valgus angles on children less than eight years old were found and increasing angles with age, worse in females, assumed to be due to the use of tighter fitting shoes (Hardy and Clapham, 1952). The African cultures do not have particularly gender-specific or tight fitting shoes, much less high heel shoes. It is difficult to say with confidence that tight-fitting shoes cause all the problems, but pointed and tight-fitting shoes certainly won't help if you already

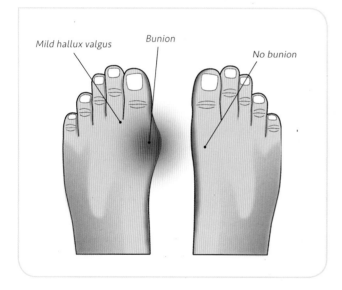

Mild hallux valgus

Bunion

No bunion

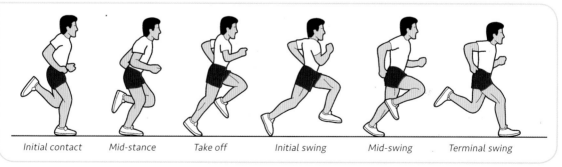

Initial contact · Mid-stance · Take off · Initial swing · Mid-swing · Terminal swing

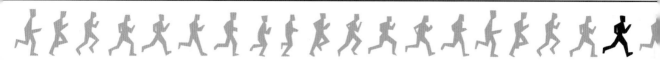

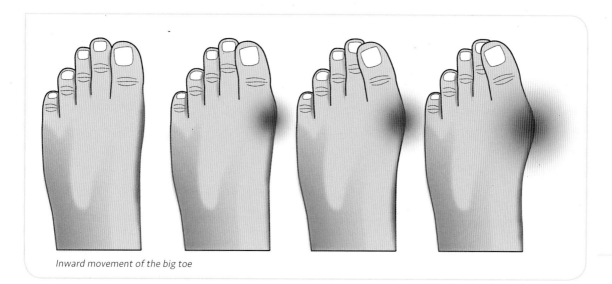

Inward movement of the big toe

have a bunion. It is well documented that females suffer much more than men, suggesting the tight-fitting shoe is relevant, but this is unsubstantiated scientifically. Perhaps ill-fitting shoes could be the prime cause, only exacerbated by biomechanics and hereditary factors.

The problems cause pain around the big toe, which becomes red, and blisters may form due to the enlarged areas rubbing against footwear.

It is at the point of the toe where the hallux limitus/rigidus becomes an issue. Hallux rigidus causes the toe to lock before full movement of the toe has been achieved. The result is abnormal knee flexion with a resultant loss of hip extension (Hall and Nester, 2004).

PROGRESSION OF THE INJURY – HALLUX VALGUS

Runners with hallux valgus are at risk of potential changes to their biomechanics. A foot plant, either heel strike or forefoot strike, can be altered if the big toe has moved from its anatomical position inward toward the second toe. The foot will no longer plant and push off the flexed big toe, but roll over its long medial edge, increasing pronation and most likely external rotation of the foot. Both of these can put additional pressure on the calf muscle, knee and hip,

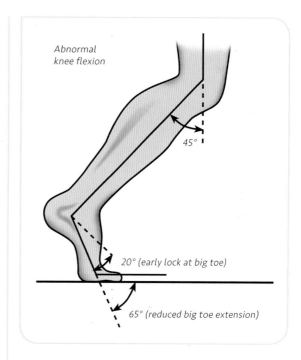

Abnormal knee flexion

45°

20° (early lock at big toe)

65° (reduced big toe extension)

leading to a whole host of additional injuries higher up the kinetic chain.

With hallux rigidus and hallux valgus, it is the stress placed on the knee and pelvis that can overload areas such as the calf, with the potential to

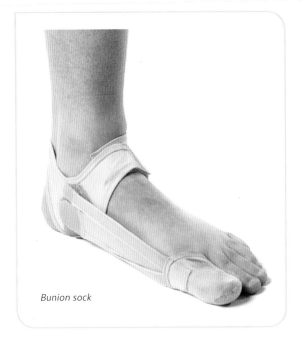

Bunion sock

cause a tear. There is significant strain placed on the plantar fascia, shin, knee, hip and even lower back. Having a rigid first toe is not however a guarantee of lower leg injury, particularly if you have a strong and well-functioning core to compensate.

SELF-ASSESSMENT

Barefoot, stand on an even surface. look down at your feet and adjust so the midlines of the feet are parallel, but with a gap between them.

Look to see if all of the toes are straight, or if the big toe is starting to angle itself toward the other four toes. If unsure, place your foot onto a clean piece of A4 paper and draw around the outline of both feet. Use this as a template to notice any change over the coming months.

If your big toe is not aligned and there is noticeable movement inward as you monitor your feet, you may well have this problem and should seek help from a physiotherapist or podiatrist.

TREATMENT

The treatment options do tend to involve surgery for hallux valgus but only once things significantly deteriorate. Before you reach this stage there are some orthotic devices that can help, just as with a Morton's neuroma. Always opt for the more expensive bespoke option rather than off-the-shelf devices as these are more effective. Wider fitting shoes are something that helps in the shorter term. The orthotic device is the treatment of choice for hallux rigidus, with a cut out for the big toe to drop down into, creating sufficient movement for the foot mechanics to be restored sufficiently.

SELF-TREATMENT

There are some slightly cumbersome items finding their way onto the market to correct hallux valgus, which are a sort of sock with individual Velcro straps that can be tightened with each passing week, to gradually bring the big toe back in line. I tried some with my patients and their feedback was simple: they didn't wear them for long enough as they found them uncomfortable. However, that isn't to say that over time this feedback won't result in an improved

design that provides comfort and functionality. It has to be said that these sorts of devices would be at optimum effectiveness when the symptoms and deformity were very mild, but how motivated are those with mild symptoms to wear such a device?

In terms of running, the main issue for both hallux conditions beyond the localized pain is the potential for hip and knee pain due to altered biomechanics. This is where a specialized set of orthotics can really help, countering the unwanted movement, thus maintaining hip and knee alignment.

Exercises to assist with any associated musculoskeletal disorders from having a hallux valgus/rigidus are Towel grabbing (strength), page 167, Calf (stretch), page 168, The clam – hip abduction/rotation (strength), page 173, Core muscles (strength), page 176 and ITB Tensor fascia latae (stretch), page 178.

WHAT TO EXPECT FROM A PHYSIOTHERAPIST

The physio or podiatrist will consider how best to maintain mechanics of the foot and minimize

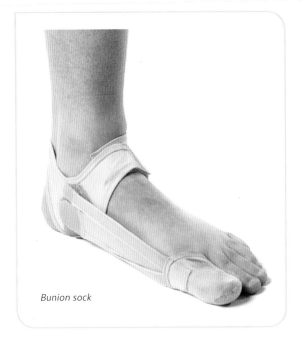

46

RUNNING FREE OF INJURIES

PRACTITIONER PROTOCOL

This presentation is highly likely to mean an onward referral for orthotic prescription. However, there are some treatment options available.

- Advice on foot mechanics and footwear
- Provide toe spacers, even if only for night wear
- Suggest one of the various splints for everyday wear such as those found at bochikun. com
- Soft tissue massage to the medial foot, mobilizations to the various joints to optimize function
- Gait analysis to look for external rotation and improper loading of the medial edge of the hallux. Could a reduction in tension of the posterior lower leg and foot mobilization reduce this mechanical stress through the hallux?
- Monitor closely over a series of well-spaced treatments.

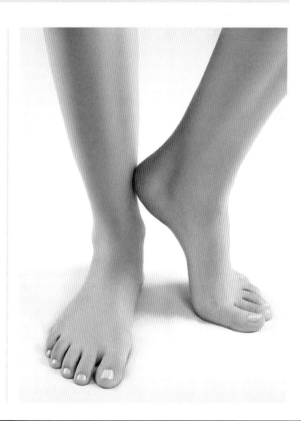

the effects higher up the kinetic chain. Orthotic devices and toe spacers are going to be the first line of treatment as well as working on the structural components involved in the alignment of ankle, knee and hip.

Advice on footwear and night splinting is to be expected in the early stages, but onward referral for surgery could be the outcome if you have left this for a long time. There are of course people I treat who are symptom-free despite quite deformed feet, with the toes crossing over and yet they have somehow maintained alignment. A physio would look to monitor their progress and only opt for surgery when necessary.

GETTING BACK TO RUNNING
This only really applies if you have required surgery. This is also dependent upon your type of surgery, as a pinned toe or fusion may reduce your ability to run and these factors would have been discussed prior to your consent for the operation. It's the ability to keep running without doing undue damage to the knee and hip that will result in a health care professional asking you to moderate your running

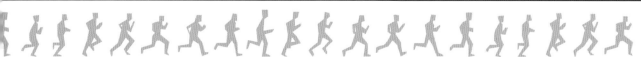

I first noticed a pain within my big toe many years ago, but I took to running late in life and so didn't realize the issues I would face once I started to exercise more. I always seemed to be sore at the big toe joint after a wedding or party at first and preferred to be barefoot or in slippers as soon as I returned home from work.

Once I reached a regular running distance of 10km per week, the pain seemed to worsen, not just when I was running but all the time. My mother had bunions, so does my elder sister and I am sure generations before me suffered.

It was a trip to the physio for some knee pain which I'd started to feel when running that picked up on the inwardly placed big toe as a potential issue. Paul was able to demonstrate with his pressure analysis software where I was placing the load through my foot when standing, walking and running, it was fascinating to learn all this about myself, if not for running, then just for everyday life.

Within four days of that assessment I had some new shiny orthotic devices for my shoes and the effect was instant. As soon as I placed my foot into my shoe with the device in place, my foot was supported, comfortable and ache-free. My knee pain hasn't come back since that day and I am happy to report that I am running pain-free for the first time since I started.

I of course still have the inward poking big toe and walking barefoot is just as it was before, but slowly I am building strength with the exercises I have been given by Paul and sense there is not only a change to my barefoot walking now, but also an improvement in my running speed.

I will admit that I had a healthy amount of scepticism, as everyone has bunions these days, yet not everyone with bunions has knee pain and then there is the cost for the orthotics, but all that faded away once I tried them for the first time. I could never put a price on how it felt running without any aches and pains for the first time.

career long-term. The choice as always is yours, but there are plenty of people who have ignored this well-meaning advice and have the knee replacement to prove it.

Metatarsal stress fracture

What is it?

A stress fracture, (known historically as a hairline fracture, although the term stress fracture is now more commonplace) is an overuse injury (Matsuda and Fukubayashi, 2015), common at the metatarsal bones in the foot, navicular (one of the tarsals) and the tibia (shin bone). Less common sites are around the hip, pelvis, sacrum and lumbar spine.

The stress fracture is developed following a repeated movement that stresses the bone, causing micro trauma from submaximal loading (Matsuda and Fukubayashi, 2015). The appearance of a stress fracture brings pain on movement, which increases as the movement is repeated, but abates with rest. The pain is characterized as being very local, for example, when palpating (touching in 'physio speak') the bone. There would be little or no pain until you hit the site of the stress fracture. Diagnosis can be improved by percussion on the bone in the form of tapping, using a tuning fork or therapeutic ultrasound waves through the bone. This will cause the pain to reproduce as the site of the stress fracture is disturbed. The metatarsals are prone to stress fracture in runners due to the forces placed through this area.

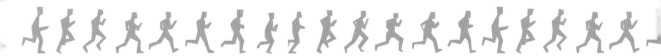

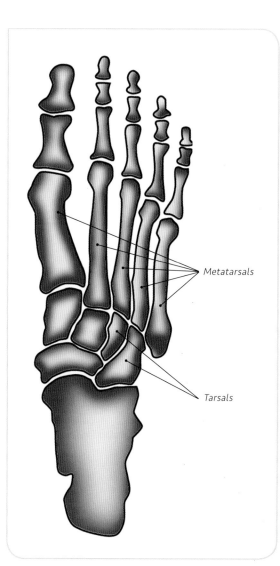

Metatarsals

Tarsals

EARLY WARNING SIGNS

- Pain on activity, at a specific site within the foot, usually over one or two metatarsals.
- Pain eases with rest
- Pain doesn't go away as activity increases, and, if anything, gets worse.

COMMON REASONS FOR INJURY

People at risk are those with:

- Poor biomechanics
- Weak glutes
- Poor foot posture
- Badly fitting footwear
- Poor running technique
- Those who increase training too quickly
- Those who try the transition from normal footwear to minimalist footwear inappropriately
- Vitamin D deficiency
- Females that train too hard and as a consequence do not menstruate
- Post-menopausal women.

The diagnosis is often missed or misdiagnosed by runners who continue on through the pain until it is unbearable. There is no shortcut to fixing this problem; regardless of your ability as a runner, you cannot speed up bone healing times.

PROGRESSION OF THE INJURY

Usually pain limits you doing any further damage, however, for those able to continue, the pain will eventually get worse as the site and spread of the

STRESSING THE POINT

There will be some repetition of information concerning fractures as one of the aims of the book, as explained in the introduction, is that the reader can dip in and out of chapters as required. So sometimes guidance on generic fractures and stress fractures will need to be repeated.

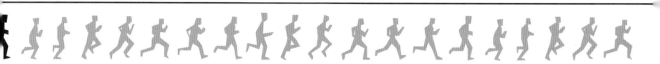

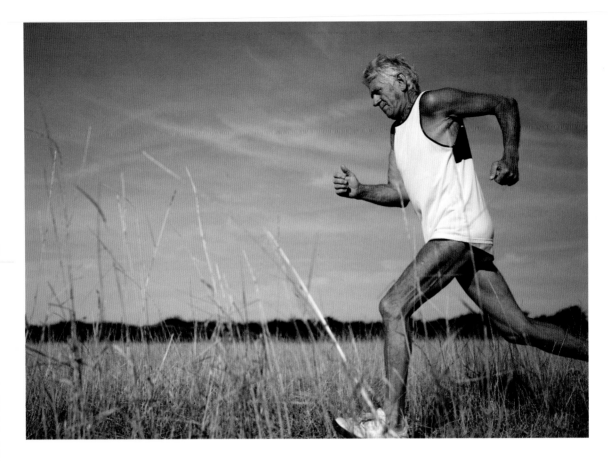

injury gets worse, prolonging your healing time once you eventually stop.

SELF-ASSESSMENT

Run your hand over the foot until you feel the area that is clearly in the most pain. Press quite firmly about three inches away from the area of pain, onto the same bone. Gradually press along the bone getting closer and closer to the site of pain. If you feel little or no pain until you are directly over the injury site, or only slightly past it, but immense pain directly over the injury, this is typical of a stress fracture.

More diffuse pain and swelling, whilst not a clear sign that this is a lesser injury, is less likely to be a stress fracture, which is a more pinpoint, very specific, acute pain.

TREATMENT

Treatment is usually rest, but in the worse cases, you could have to wear an aircast boot (a boot that is pumped full of air to support and protect the limb against impact) for six weeks. Physiotherapists can usually diagnose this quite effectively. Stress fractures are only visible when they start to heal as you can see the bone that is laid down for healing (callus) around the fracture site. Therefore, X-rays should be taken at least four weeks after the onset of symptoms. If the X-ray does not show the fracture, an MRI or CT scan may be required.

SELF-TREATMENT

Rest! The main point is that you absolutely need to rest. The key to recovery is adhering to the period set out by your clinician. Usually it's a

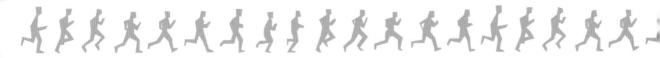

six-week rest period, but that doesn't mean you can just drop straight back into running at the end of the six weeks.

Exercises to assist the smooth return to a programme and to keep up some lower limb conditioning use the following exercises from the appendix: The clam – hip abduction/rotation (strength), page 173, Hamstrings (strength), page 174, Glute activation (strength), page 175, Core muscles (strength), page 176, Swiss ball abduction in side plank, page 180 and Bridge, page 184.

WHAT TO EXPECT FROM A PHYSIOTHERAPIST

For assessment purposes, your physio will listen to you as this usually provides all the clues needed to make the diagnosis. They would then put some ultrasound gel on the 'good' foot, and slowly move the handheld scanner back and forth over the metatarsals, expecting (and explaining) that there shouldn't be any pain. They will then do the same thing on the sore foot and positive diagnosis is pain over the site of the injury, as therapeutic ultrasound will produce sound waves that unsettle the stress fracture and cause pain, it doesn't cause pain through any healthy bone or other soft tissues. X-rays are not very effective until at least four weeks after the original fracture so MRI scans are used to confirm the diagnosis. From there an orthopaedic boot will be worn for six weeks and in extremely bad cases, crutches need to be used as well.

GETTING BACK TO RUNNING

I have spent many an hour working out return-to-running programmes for athletes who are starting back after a stress fracture. The focus is on cross training initially with 80–90% of your time doing activities other than running. During the phase of injury you can aqua jog to your heart's content and, if you can get to access them, there are expensive anti-gravity treadmills that will allow you to spend some time running, but with as little as a few per cent of your body weight being transferred through your body. Under close scrutiny you can develop the loading through the foot over a painstakingly long period.

PRACTITIONER PROTOCOL

Use your ultrasound machine to help with the assessment. Turn it up to a high, continuous setting and see if there is pain over the site of injury. If unsure, then send for an MRI scan where possible.

Treatment will depend upon severity, but for completeness, opt for non-weight bearing until you have a firm diagnosis.

- Speed recovery with an orthopaedic boot for six weeks
- Use the assessment session to look at general strength and conditioning of the runner, check for core strength, glute activation, hamstring equality and hip flexor tightness
- Set a programme around your findings with home exercises that do not load the injured foot.
- Set aqua jogging sessions and a full series of strength and conditioning exercises specific to running to ensure that the runner can return to full fitness as quickly as possible post recovery.

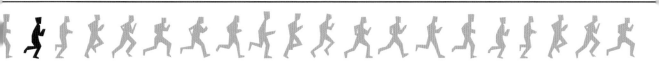

Typically, you need to aqua jog for the six weeks you are in a protective boot and then you can start back on the cross trainer, eventually decreasing your time on this in favour of increasing bouts of running on soft ground. Your final transition will be back to the track or pavement.

CLIENT STORY: SARAH, 24

It was during my training for a marathon that I started to feel a pain in my right foot, which didn't really concern me at first as, to be honest, everything was hurting and I assumed it was just the way I was going to feel for the next 16 weeks of the programme I'd downloaded from the Internet. I had decided to run the marathon for a charity and had started to fundraise so the thought of getting injured when I didn't really have that long to train was awful to me. About a week after I started to feel my foot ache, I decided to rest for a few days, whereupon the foot did actually feel quite a lot better – pain-free in fact. Having missed so much training already I tried to do slightly more than the programme suggested in an attempt to catch up.

On a long run, I noticed my foot starting to hurt more and more and eventually had to stop. The pain got even worse after I stopped and I was really very uncomfortable. I walked home, stopping regularly as my foot felt like it was throbbing and I was clearly limping.

At home I iced the foot and decided to rest it for a few more days and take some anti-inflammatories. The pain was once again much more manageable but this time it didn't go away. I feel silly now, but despite the pain I decided I had to train as I really wanted to make it around the marathon course. Within just a few hundred metres of my run, it was clear I wasn't going anywhere and I limped back home. This time however I searched the Internet for someone to take a look at my foot. Seeing the website for Physio&Therapy and the tweet from Paula Radcliffe saying that Paul had fixed her ankle meant I knew who to call.

Within minutes of being in the clinic, Paul had broken the news to me that he thought I had a stress

fracture – he had barely looked at my foot at this stage. It wasn't what I wanted to hear. He used an ultrasonic device on my good foot and I felt nothing, but he warned me that if he was right and I had a stress fracture then it would hurt on my injured foot as the waves would unsettle the bone injury. I felt the pain instantly and knew that he was right. I was sent for an MRI scan because the X-rays don't show up stress fractures very well in the early stages of injury. The scan confirmed that I had a stress fracture in my metatarsal bone next to my big toe and I was placed in a big boot to stop me injuring my foot any more. Six weeks rest and only 12 weeks until the marathon and my dreams of running the race were dashed, it just couldn't be done.

It was Paul who explained that I just needed to refocus and suggested running a marathon later in the year. He told me the Dublin marathon was great and not until October so that gave me plenty of time. He joked that you can also enter on the day, so I didn't have to make my mind up until I felt I was ready. This was a huge relief and I was able to explain to my sponsors that I had a change of plan and they all kept to their pledges for my charity.

The road to recovery was fairly simple really: I just had to rest for six weeks. Paul gave me all sorts of other exercises to do following an assessment to seek out my areas of weakness. I was also told to try aqua jogging, although I have to admit that I didn't get on well with that, so I opted to just do the rehab and leave running alone for a while.

The good news is that after all that I had a full recovery and with the extra rehabilitation and personalized programme over a much longer period of time I ran the Dublin marathon in 4hrs 24 minutes and consider that a total success.

The process is a long one but, if rushed, can be followed by a further eight weeks back in the boot and a slower return to running. I have seen over-eager athletes lose a whole year through early return over and over again, unable to follow the more cautious advice from their physio.

But why did the stress fracture occur in the first instance? If there is a clear history of overuse, ramping training levels too high, incorrect footwear choice or a confirmed starting point, then perhaps just the recovery as outlined is sufficient. However, there is often an underlying mechanical cause which needs investigating and I favour spending time with a piece of equipment called Footscan.

Footscan became popular in running shops in the 1990s as it helped determine what footwear choice the customer should opt for, demonstrating pronation and supination and pressure transference in colour-coded real-time technology. Being able to look closely at the micro-data contained within the system, you can see where pressure is being produced at high levels and how the foot has to absorb unnecessary levels over certain structures within it.

The technology has advanced and today the use of Footscan is commonplace in physio clinics to identify the aspects of the gait cycle that a physio is unable to see with their trained eye alone. It's not the sole assessment tool, but physios like myself use this equipment to build a picture of the patient. Footscan can now be used in conjunction with a 3D printer to produce orthotic insoles. These insoles can then be tested on delivery and before and after images compared.

I am happy to use this equipment on my clients and in many cases to produce orthotic insoles for the common issues I see.

Cuboid syndrome

What is it?

The cuboid is one of the small bones that make up the tarsal bones of the foot. The cuboid is just by the base of the fourth and fifth metatarsals. It is believed that it can become immobile and potentially move microscopically from its true location due to acute traumatic injury or repeated movements such as running. This can cause significant pain, usually at the site of the cuboid, the lateral ankle and also along the 4th metatarsal. Cuboid syndrome is often overlooked and misdiagnosed as an ankle sprain or stress fracture.

EARLY WARNING SIGNS

It is important to reiterate that for this injury the early warning signs mimic a great deal of other injuries, such as a sprained ankle or stress fracture. It is very difficult to decide on a specific pattern that would determine this individual injury. The main symptoms to look out for are:

- Pain along the fourth metatarsal
- Lateral ankle pain
- Foot arch pain
- Sudden onset of pain without knowing the specific cause.

Diagnosing cuboid syndrome is as much about discounting other injuries as it is a formal diagnosis.

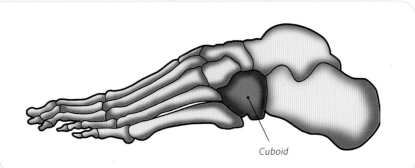

Cuboid

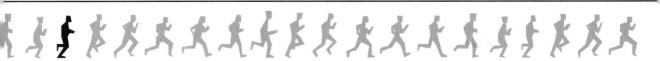

As the symptoms correlate with those of a stress fracture, the use of therapeutic ultrasound along the fourth metatarsal to see if it causes acute pain is a good indicator that it is not a stress fracture, however it doesn't diagnose cuboid syndrome.

COMMON REASONS FOR INJURY

It can be quite common to experience cuboid syndrome at the same time as an ankle sprain or after repeated ankle sprains further complicating diagnosis. As the ankle inverts into the sprain, the muscle peroneus longus (responsible for eversion and dorsiflexion of the foot) pulls sharply to try to correct the foot position. The tendon for peroneus longus sits in a groove on the underside of the cuboid. This groove in the cuboid facilitates a direction change in the tendon, before its journey under the foot to the attachment at the first metatarsal. This forceful contraction with an ankle sprain pulls the cuboid awkwardly and can cause the adjacent bones to jam tightly together, which means the changes are too small to see on X-ray or even a MRI scan.

PROGRESSION OF THE INJURY

I have seen a client with this issue go undiagnosed for 12 weeks. They were sent from consultant to consultant and placed in an orthopaedic boot for over six weeks. The pain is so intense that patients prefer not to put their foot down, resorting to crutches and staying home from work in severe cases. It simply doesn't seem to get better, worse if anything. Yet the disaster in all this is that it is usually very simple to resolve.

SELF-ASSESSMENT

This is very difficult to self-diagnose. The majority of people I have seen with this have visited a great number of practitioners and been told that nothing was discovered on X-ray or MRI scan. If you are struggling with ankle pain, or particularly pain that radiates along your fourth metatarsal without any other cause, consider this as a potential diagnosis.

Run your hands along the little toe, then along the metatarsal bone. Towards the ankle, there is a clearly defined end to the metatarsal with a little dip in towards the foot just past the end of the fifth metatarsal, but before the ankle bone that sticks out.

With your fingertip grip underneath the foot with your thumb on top of the lateral foot. You should be able to feel a bone between your fingers. If this bone is particularly painful when compared to your uninjured side, consider cuboid syndrome and seek treatment from a physiotherapist.

TREATMENT

When considering cuboid syndrome as a primary diagnosis, the treatment which is an adjustment of the cuboid (known as the 'black snake whip') brings almost immediate relief, which in itself confirms the diagnosis.

SELF-TREATMENT

Use exercises Towel grabbing (strength), page 167, Soleus (stretch), page 168, Toe raises (strength), page 169, The clam – hip abduction/rotation (strength), page 173 and Core muscles (strength), page 176 to assist with the overall conditioning of the area and kinetic chain.

WHAT TO EXPECT FROM A PHYSIOTHERAPIST

Physiotherapists can mobilize the cuboid, providing almost instant relief. After the mobilization, the physio will usually tape the foot, so as to try to keep the cuboid tightly bound. A series of treatments may well be necessary depending upon the duration of the injury and the biomechanics of the individual, using orthosis to balance and stabilize the foot. Calf stretches are prescribed initially before building onto strengthening exercises once pain-free.

GETTING BACK TO RUNNING

If you are able to move relatively pain-free and can tolerate the tape, then a gradual return to normal activity can begin.

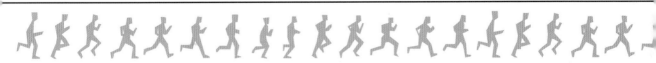

PRACTITIONER PROTOCOL

In the absence of any other diagnosis, check the cuboid for pain and mobility. If there is significantly more pain on the injured side when the cuboid is palpated, try an adjustment to see if symptoms are improved.

- Warm up all surrounding tissues with some soft tissue work
- Apply a grade 2 AP (anterior to poterior) and PA (posterior to anterior) force through the cuboid and reassess
- Apply grade 3, then 4, and reassess at each stage
- Grade 5 manipulate the cuboid (e.g. black snake whip) then reassess
- SSTM to the peroneus longus to reduce pull through the plantar aspect of cuboid
- Apply kinesiology tape around the cuboid, in a full wrap, twice around the foot, leaving no tension in an area away from the cuboid for maintenance of fluid dynamics
- If the patient is pain-free following treatment, tell them to rest two days and attempt a short rehab run. If pain remains, continue to treat in this way until pain-free before commencement of rehabilitation running schedule.

Rehab runs to consist of 5 x 3 minutes with gastrocnemius and soleus stretches.

CLIENT STORY: ROSS, 28

I had been doing triathlons for the past two years when I decided to take the step up to Olympic distance from sprint. This by its nature meant more training was needed in all three disciplines.

As the running intensity increased I began experiencing some mild discomfort in my foot, however, I thought it was nothing of concern. Race day came and the run was on uneven ground. Half way round the 10k run my foot was in agony. The pain in the outer bit of my arch of my left foot was something I had never experienced before. I'm not really sure how I managed to cope but I ran through the rest of the race and finished it. However, after the race I could not put any weight on it and had to walk on my tiptoes to take the pain away.

Paul was recommended to me by one of my friends from triathlon. At the first session I attended, Paul was able to diagnose the issue within two minutes of me stepping in: cuboid syndrome. Paul manipulated my foot which instantly allowed me to walk normally and the pain had subsided. He then recommended some strength building exercise and strapped my foot up.

Paul also recommended I stop running for a few weeks while the area healed. I was still able to swim and bike without issue, and after three sessions I was able to start running again and gradually start building up to my usual distances.

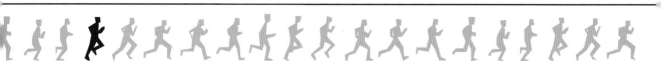

CHAPTER 2

THE ANKLE

There are two main joints in the ankle, the subtalar joint found between the heel bone (calcaneus) and the talus bone, and the talo crural, or ankle mortise joint. Both can have their own issues; as with any joint, they can become inflamed and also have reduced movement, in turn reducing the function of the whole foot and ankle complex.

We will be looking at the following common injuries:

- Subtalar joint and talo crural joint pain
- Ankle ligament sprain
- Achilles tendinopathy.

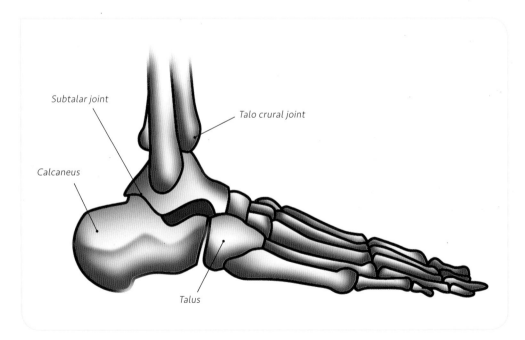

Subtalar joint

Talo crural joint

Calcaneus

Talus

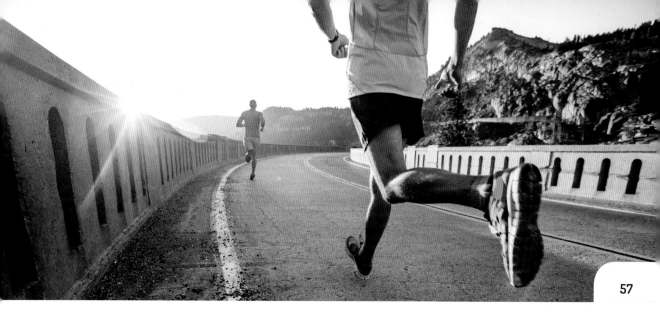

Subtalar joint and talo crural (mortise) joint pain

What is it?

The subtalar joint sits just under the talus, and the talo crural (mortise) joint is just above. The movements around these two joints provide all the dorsiflexion and plantarflexion (mortise joint) and inversion/eversion (sub talar joint), as well as abduction and adduction making the ankle a highly mobile joint. Supination and pronation comes from the tarsal and metatarsal bones in the foot.

The ankle joints themselves can cause pain when the joint surfaces are affected. Osteoarthritis can cause small bony spurs called osteophytes to grow and these can cause anterior ankle impingement. Ankle impingement is caused by repeated micro trauma breaking down the articular cartilage or capsule that surrounds the ankle. The repeated trauma required for this injury results in the nickname athlete's ankle or footballer's ankle. The pain is usually anteriolateral (at the front and to the outside) or anteriomedial (at the front and to the inside).

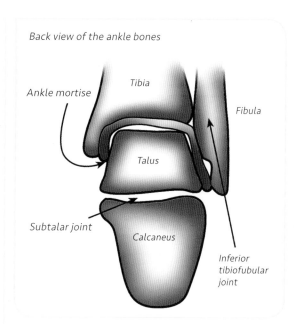

Back view of the ankle bones

Ankle mortise

Tibia

Fibula

Talus

Subtalar joint

Calcaneus

Inferior tibiofubular joint

EARLY WARNING SIGNS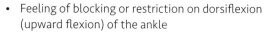

- Pain in the anterior ankle joint
- Feeling of blocking or restriction on dorsiflexion (upward flexion) of the ankle
- Pain on ankle movements
- Swelling around the anterior ankle joint
- Tenderness on ankle joint movements.

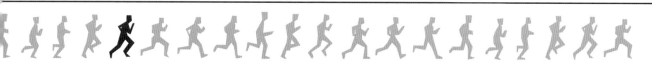

COMMON REASONS FOR INJURY

- Those who have experienced repeated ankle sprains
- Those with a chronic instability of the ankle
- Poorly fitting shoes
- Increasing exercise
- Sports such as football, rugby, netball and basketball.

PROGRESSION OF THE INJURY

Ankle pain and instability can become chronic and the joint surfaces suffer due to wear and tear making pain and early onset osteoarthritis a common progression. Inflammation can be present over a long period of time, changing the fluid dynamics of the joint and leading to long-term instability and pain.

SELF-ASSESSMENT

There are no diagnostic tests as such, but you should compare range of movement from one ankle to another.

Sit with your feet outstretched, and visually measure the amount you can turn your feet inward and outwards, also rotate inwards and outwards. Assess the amount you can point your toes (plantar flexion) and then pull them up (dorsiflexion).

See how closely each movement mirrors the other, and look for obvious differences. If, for example, you are unable to dorsiflex your left foot, then there may be an issue with one of your ankle joints and you should seek confirmation from your physiotherapist.

TREATMENT

I am not always a fan of ankle surgery unless absolutely necessary. The opportunity for physiotherapy and orthotics to be tried first is always my goal, however some simple procedures such as keyhole surgery to remove an osteophyte are fairly simple and will help significantly. Also an injection to the ankle joint or either steroid or ostenil can reduce inflammation and pain. Once the

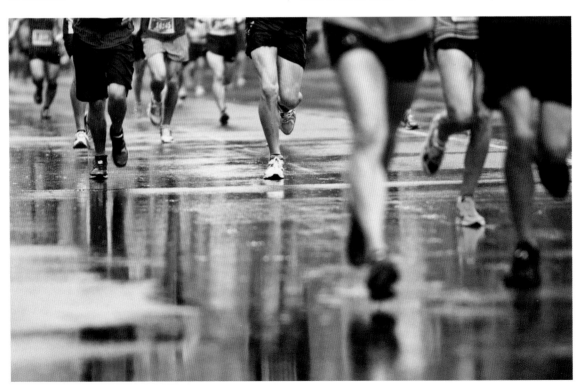

PRACTITIONER PROTOCOL

Assess the ankle as you would do normally, but look specifically for areas of instability or tension during the range of movement as this is where you can have most immediate effect.

- Soft tissue massage to the lower leg to warm up with frictions around the ankle joints and reassess function
- Mobilize the ankle joint responsible for the lack of movement and reassess function
- Mobilize the tarsal joints and reassess function
- Make detailed notes for each stage and record the relative changes between session results
- Where there is laxity or instability use kinesiology tape to support only that area, whilst providing strengthening exercises for the muscles in question
- Move onto balance work and then balance cushions and BOSU®-based gym work
- A small trampette can be very useful for more dynamic training, although inexpensive, they are not always available
- Return to run rehab should involve multi-directional hopping and agility drills similar to those used for football or rugby rehabilitation.

injection has been administered, full ankle stability and range of movement exercises should be the goal to increase movement and reduce instability.

SELF-TREATMENT
Work on mobility and strength. The ankle requires a huge amount of strength and when working optimally (Baltich *et al.*, 2015) has a vast array of available movement when combined with the foot joints. (This is largely the same as the ankle ligament sprains in the following section.)

Perform the following exercises: Peroneals–ankle eversion (strength), page 170, Single leg balance, page 171 and Side step with squat (strength), page 179.

WHAT TO EXPECT FROM A PHYSIOTHERAPIST
Once the diagnosis has been obtained a physiotherapist can mobilize the joint using specialist techniques to glide and slide the joint surfaces to maintain or restore optimal movement. This isn't limited to the joint in question, as often the injured joint owes its overload to the loss of movement in neighbouring joints in the first place; a physiotherapist can step in not only to treat the symptom but to tackle the underlying cause as well.

You may find that there is a great deal of soft tissue work surrounding the area, and pressure being placed through joints as far away as the knee, sometimes with audible, pain-free clicks.

Expect some fairly challenging exercises. As a runner, some of the exercises should be based around the sort of positions you find yourself in during a run, whilst achieving the work around the ankle that is required.

GETTING BACK TO RUNNING
The timeline can often be muddled depending on a variety of factors, such as those who have injections, or those who have manipulations, taped and not taped, etc. For the majority of people, expect a slow

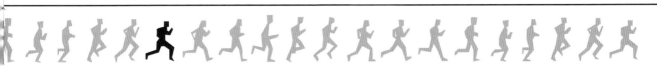

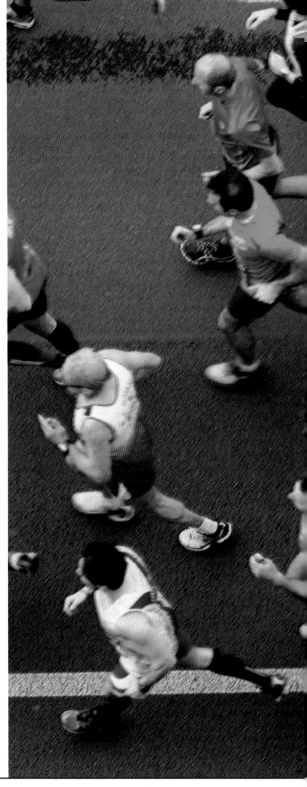

GRADE 2

Grade 2 ligament injuries mean damage to over 25% of the body of the ligament through to about 75%.

Very painful, with lots more swelling. Often the eventual swelling will cover an area similar to that of a trainer sock, taking up most of the lateral foot, around the ankle and across the top of the foot as well. These are extremely painful when first done, make walking difficult and a common reason for people to attend A&E straight after the sprain expecting there to be a fracture.

GRADE 3

Grade 3 ligament injuries have caused a full thickness rupture of the ligament. These bruise like a full sock, with everything going black and blue, and are typically painful, but there are cases of very little pain at all after the initial incident has subsided. The reason is that the ligament has snapped altogether and therefore the remaining fibres are not being stressed. Cases where there is a full rupture of ATFL (grade 3) but no involvement of CFL or PTFL are often less painful than a grade 2 sprain to the ankle.

The ligament is made up of collagen. Collagen has three main types of fibre: types 1, 2 and 3. Type 1 collagen is the primary connective tissue in the body and makes up ligaments and tendons and can be thought of as mature collagen. Type 3 collagen is what's created after injury; scar tissue is largely formed of type 3 collagen. Type 2 collagen is found in many of the joint surfaces as a structure known as hyaline cartilage.

Collagen is found everywhere from the skin to artery walls, in bone as well as in muscle. Collagen is made up of a variety of different cells, the boss of these being the macrophage or director cell. The macrophage decides how much and in what proportion the fibroblasts (the cells that lay down new collagen) are released. Fibroblasts make up the majority of the cell matrix and are integral to the repair process.

Mast cells are the cells most associated with inflammation and are part of our immune system. When we sprain an ankle, it's important to realize that the chosen treatments are aimed at these

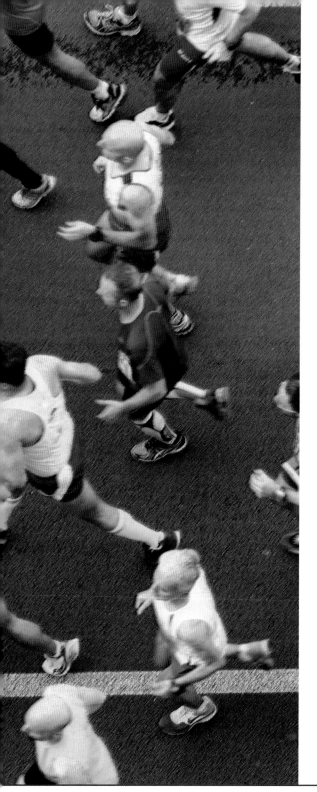

cells, to develop, or reduce, production of each to best facilitate healing. For example, your body does a great job in producing lots of great work early on in the injury, so if manual physiotherapy is used too early, it can unsettle the process. The use of steroid injections actually inhibits the production of macrophages, so it would be counterproductive to use this as a form of therapy in the early stages, despite its ability to reduce inflammation. The same goes for ibuprofen and other non-steroidal anti-inflammatories, which reduce collagen synthesis as well.

In fact, the body is so good at early repair that within the first 12 hours of injury there are signs of early capillary formation. The inflammatory phase peaks in the first four days. This may mean that the use of Rest, Ice, Compression, and Elevation (R.I.C.E.) may no longer be the most effective treatment. Simply allow your body time to do what it's designed to do for the initial 72 hours as nothing has been found to be an improvement on the body's natural forces. However, if there is pain and inflammation present, until we glean more scientific evidence to the contrary, I still advocate using R.I.C.E. as first line treatment, but without using anti-inflammatory medications for at least 72 hours.

EARLY WARNING SIGNS

This is an acute injury, so there are no early warning signs as such. The issue is to determine if you have sprained your ankle and to what grade. Use the information above to assist with the grading process.

- Immediate pain from acute injury
- Immediate swelling
- If severe you will be unable to load through the leg
- The swelling will start at the lateral ankle bone but could spread to a larger area.

COMMON REASONS FOR INJURY

- Twisting of ankle whilst turning or landing awkwardly
- Slipping off a kerb or sidewalk

- Uneven surface or unseen holes causing the ankle to slip into a void unexpectedly.

SELF-ASSESSMENT

Everyone's pain is subjective and therefore not a great measure of what level of injury you have sustained, but assuming you haven't broken your ankle, the following will loosely assist you with the grade of ankle sprain.

Range of movement when compared to the uninjured side is:

- The same – probably grade 1
- Laxity increased slightly – probably grade 2
- Laxity significantly increased – probably grade 3.

Pain levels after the initial period of acute pain is:

- Bearable – grade 1
- Extremely high – grade 2
- Ranging from none to unbearable – grade 3.

Despite the all-inclusive nature of the third option, the combination of pain scale and range of movement can lead you to the correct diagnosis.

Another way to diagnose is a day or so later when the bruising is fully developed:

- Golf ball size swelling and mild bruising – grade 1
- Significant bruising around the immediate ankle and a line along the lateral foot – grade 2
- Bruising that could be mistaken for a sock – grade 3.

TREATMENT

Once the 72 hours post-acute injury are over, it's time for physiotherapy. A physiotherapist would be looking to stimulate the ligament with some transverse frictions. The deep pressure of the fingertips, moving backward and forwards over the ligament, works initially to numb the area of pain, in much the same way your mother would rub your knee when you bumped it. This neural overload means that the brain doesn't feel the pain

KINESIOLOGY TAPE

I am an avid fan of kinesiology tape and in fact got into a spot of bother just before the 2012 London Olympic Games when I was quoted in the *Guardian* as saying 'it's the best thing to happen to physiotherapy for 10 years.' My actual words were that I had been using zinc oxide tape for 10 years and I felt that kinesiology tape was better for many of my regular applications.

So why do I like kinesiology tape? It's not because it's supposed to attach to the muscle and aid contraction, and it's not because it's supposed to help with lymphatic drainage – as I can no more see these effects than I can see any reason for the range of colours. What I do see with kinesiology tape is a product that enables you to moderate movement in a part of the joint whilst maintaining a neighbouring and desirable movement. The old-fashioned zinc oxide tape would block all movement as it had no 'give' in it whatsoever and often only remained effective for the duration of the warm-up. Kinesiology tape can endure swimming as well as sweat and will remain effective for about four days on average.

any more. Patients often report that the physio has 'slipped off the ligament' so quick is the reaction. Then a few deeper, more effective sweeps can be performed. This process is designed to stimulate the

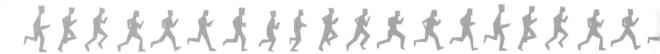

macrophages (director cells) into laying down more fibroblasts (repair cells).

Ultrasound (US) therapy is believed to work on the mast cells' degranulation which is part of the healing process (Baker *et al.*, 2001). The degranulation of mast cells, releases a substance called histamine into the tissue which is believed to increase local blood flow. US therapy has come under scrutiny in recent years (Rantanen, *et al.*, 1999) and it is more common today to use soft tissue work and the newly fashionable brightly coloured kinesiology tape, as seen on many top sports people.

You can treat an ATFL with deep transverse frictions, and tape across the ligament to reduce inversion of the ankle, but maintain the plantar and dorsiflexion capabilities and the ability to evert the ankle. This is extremely therapeutic and offers a patient better treatment.

SELF-TREATMENT

You need to gradually build up the surface instability that you work from when doing your exercises.

PRACTITIONER PROTOCOL

Assess the ankle for comparison between left and right. Check for any malleolus pain, with pain along the distal 6 cm of the posterior edge of the tibia or fibula. If present, check to see if they bear weight for four steps immediately after the injury. If the above tests are positive then refer for an X-ray for suspected fracture.

If the above tests are negative then check range of movement. Range of movement when compared to the uninjured side is:

- The same – probably grade 1
- Laxity increased slightly – probably grade 2
- Laxity significantly increased – probably grade 3.

Treatment then consists of:

- Within the first 72 hours, only R.I.C.E. and kinesiology tape
- Begin to gently mobilise the soft tissues after 72 hours with light massage and reapply the tape
- Gentle transverse frictions can be applied at this stage
- Gradually increase the depth of the treatments over the coming weeks
- Continue to tape the ankle and teach the patient how to apply the tape themselves if necessary between visits
- Once pain is manageable, start eccentric exercises for the ankle, gentle balance work and gait assessment
- Build the balance work and strength through to concentric, full range and through to hopping and jumping exercises
- Agility training prior to return to play.

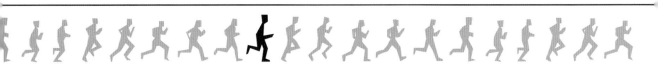

The injured ligament will be getting support from neighbouring muscles such as the peroneals and exercises can be directed towards building up these key ankle muscles (see page 170).

Here are the exercises to help with recovery: Calf (stretch), page 168, Soleus (stretch), page 168, Peroneals–ankle eversion (strength), page 170, Single leg balance, page 171, depending upon ability, Clock lunges, page 185 and Multi-direction hopping, page 186.

If the pain is still quite severe, try starting with the slightly easier form of balance exercise as described in the Foot and Ankle proprioception box on page 18.

WHAT TO EXPECT FROM A PHYSIOTHERAPIST

A physiotherapist should briefly inform you of what has occurred and explain the injury process aiding your understanding of pain modulation. You would then receive some soft tissue treatment to the ankle which is largely dependent upon the stage of the injury, however, deep transverse frictions over the injured ligament(s) is the best form of treatment.

Tape is used to great effect, so watch how your ankle is being taped as you may well be instructed to reapply this yourself between treatments. It is important that you continue to tape or use a support on your ATFL sprains for months in light of the latest research. In addition, extremely rigorous strength and conditioning programmes should be provided by the physio for you to do at home, involving lots of balance work and sport-specific movements to ensure the same injury does not repeat itself. Balance and proprioception are the buzz words in ankle rehabilitation.

GETTING BACK TO RUNNING

With a grade 1 sprain, there is a very short gap of up to two weeks before you can return to running with

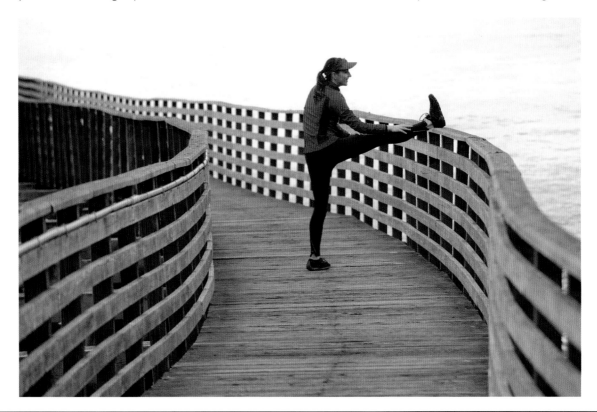

I have been a recreational runner for several years, with a typical week consisting of approximately 20 miles made up of hill training, efforts on the flat and a long, slow run, having never suffered any major injuries at all.

One evening I decided to go for a tempo run including a downhill section in a local forest. The sun was shining, the forest was filled with the beautiful smell of pine trees and I felt invincible ... until my left foot was taken from underneath me with the help of a hidden tree root! My foot bent sharply inwards and made a loud cracking noise, like someone clapping their hands. I felt instant, intense pain that increased over the coming minutes. A&E beckoned and on removing my trainer and sock I could see the outside of my ankle had started to swell badly. An X-Ray showed no breakages and I was sent home with a crepe bandage, anti-inflammatory pills, pain killers and crutches, with the advice of rest, ice, compression and elevation (R.I.C.E.) for at least the next 72 hours.

Having been a client of Paul's in the past I made an appointment to find out his diagnosis and the best way forward. On examination he told me it was a Grade 2 strain of the ATFL and at present was too swollen to work on, so suggested coming back in three days time and to stop taking the anti-inflammatories because my body was far better at naturally helping my foot initially and this specific type of medication was slowing the process down.

In the coming weeks the swelling started to go down and the bruising came out, but being injured and not being able to do any sport really hit me hard. You start to wonder: 'will I ever run again?' At that point I would have given anything just to be able to walk without being in pain.

Paul used kinesiology tape on my ankle, which gave me the support and confidence I needed to put weight on it again and start some easy bike sessions in the gym. This then progressed onto short cross-trainer sessions, always being careful that the following day my ankle hadn't swollen up again, which would have meant I had pushed it too hard.

Each week I had a series of treatments that included soft tissue work around the ankle, with some specific back and forth work with his fingertips over the most painful part of the ligament as well as continually taping the ankle.

Four weeks after the accident, after strapping up my ankle, I was able to walk for two miles pain and crutch free – a real milestone. I could have cried!

I continued with physio, including some gentle exercises for the ankle, which initially meant just holding my ankle in a certain position against a resistance band for a few seconds at a time. Being committed to getting better I did these religiously. At the six-week point, again whilst strapped up, another milestone was reached – 5km on the gym treadmill – and I started to believe that being a runner again might just be possible.

Before I'd got injured I'd signed up for the Coniston half marathon which was eight weeks after the accident, so the big question I needed answering by Paul was: 'Could I take part in the race, even if it meant walking all of it?'

The answer was just what I wanted to hear – as long as my ankle was taped, I would be fine to take part in the event, slow jogging on the flat and downhill sections but walking the uphill sections as the flexibility on my ankle still wasn't 100%, which made uphill running more painful. Race day came and I completed it in under three hours, which considering the hilly route, my fitness and the lack of training I had been able to do, proved what a major part physio had played in getting me to this stage so soon after my accident.

After the race, I continued with the physio, doing more rigorous exercises, including multidirectional hopping, lunges and standing on various unstable cushions to work on my balance. And a year on, I have just completed my first Ultra in the Lake District, with nothing more than a very small blister for an injury! I am in no doubt that the physio I received back then helped to repair my ligaments, reduce any scar tissue as a result of the accident and strengthen my ankle to make me the stronger runner that I am today.

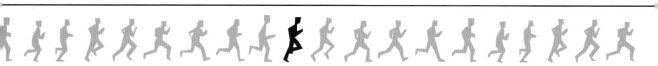

tape and alongside your exercises (please do not do strengthening exercises for your ankle before you go out for a run, you will exhaust the very muscles you need to work hard throughout the run and increase your risk of further injury). You will notice a lack of stretching in the treatment for Achilles, because stretching has been shown to irritate the tendon, which is why I like to include lots of soft tissue to the calf muscles during treatment.

Grade 2 ankle sprains are much more complex and you will be out of action for approximately six–eight weeks.

With a Grade 3 ligament injury where surgery has been necessary or immobilization in a cast, returning to running may be delayed for a long time; individual cases vary, but the ligament will be fragile for months. The decision to return to running after this means answering the question, 'does the benefit outweigh the risk?' Could you stand the heartache of re-injury after a long break from training versus waiting another week?

Achilles tendinopathy

What is it?

Achilles tendinopathy is one of the most common issues I see as a running specialist. The Achilles is the tendon that attaches the gastrocnemius and soleus muscles (known together as the calf muscles) to the calcaneus (heel bone). The Achilles is such a common area for runners to injure that only the knee can knock it off the top of the injury leader board. The pain felt at the Achilles is noticed more as stiffness initially, first thing in the morning. Patients complain of this stiffness becoming worse in the morning as the weeks progress, but do not seek help at this stage because the stiffness and pain wear off quite quickly. It's only when the pain starts to influence their running do they present to clinic in search of some answers.

The Internet is such a useful tool for runners these days, so most people come having attempted calf raises already. They may well have sought help at the local running shop and been prescribed heel raises, which will have helped a little initially but only seem to compound the problem within a short space of time.

EARLY WARNING SIGNS

- Pain in the Achilles tendon, mid portion
- Pain specifically at the insertion of the Achilles into the heel bone
- Tight calf muscles
- Loss of dorsiflexion (lifting toes up)
- Pain for the first few steps in the morning in the Achilles
- Stiffness in the calf and Achilles first thing in the morning.

COMMON REASONS FOR INJURY
The injury cause is largely unknown, despite several Internet articles suggesting that it's down to poorly fitting shoes, bad running technique or, my personal bugbear, due to over-pronation. The fact is, we just don't know what the main cause is for developing Achilles pain. It seems fairly certain that it is unlikely to be just one clearly defined cause. What we do know is that the tendon itself breaks down. When it becomes injured it affects the collagen fibres that make up the tendon and this causes stiffness and pain. The fibres have a short-lived period of inflammation and then what's left is a sort of watery soup that causes disruption to the fibres, which creates the common bump seen on the distal ⅓ of the tendon.

There are two types of Achilles injury, the more acute 'reactive tendon' which is as result of an over-loading of the tendon in some way, and there is a degenerative tendon where the issues have been there for a long time. A degenerative tendon can be 'managed' by careful use, such as sticking to your known training pattern, avoiding hills etc., however step up your training slightly on a degenerative tendon and the health parts may overload and you now have a reactive (more acute) injury to these areas. The result is pain and loss of function.

When an Achilles tendon (or any tendonopathy for that matter) becomes damaged, part of the

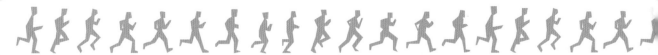

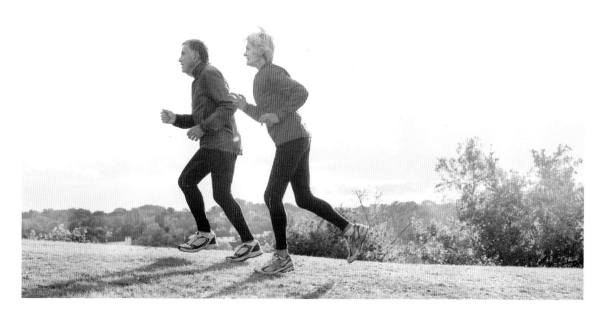

healing process is neovascularisation whereby blood vessels work their way into the tendon along with nerve fibres in an attempt to heal the tendon. This blood supply can be seen within the fibres of an injured Achilles using a dopla.

During the acute phase (although these injuries are chronic in nature there has to be a start point of injury which we refer to as acute or onset of injury) the additional fluid within the structure creates an opportunity for blood vessels to work their way into the tendon from the fat pad just anterior to the Achilles. This blood supply can be seen within the fibres of chronic Achilles injury using a dopla ultrasound scanner, which shows the vessels as red and blue dots pulsing on the screen (blood in and blood out) thus confirming the stage of injury and directing rehabilitation.

Early stage management of an Achilles tendon injury is the key to success. For those patients who present early, on first signs of soreness, it is highly likely that just the outer layer of the Achilles will be inflamed, known as the paratendon. The paratendon can become inflamed and irritated causing similar symptoms to a full-blown Achilles tendinopathy.

The Achilles itself has a very short-lived period of inflammation, if any at all. The breakdown of tendon fibres occurs for a large number of reasons, not all of them known to us. Of course we can make assumptions such as the ones you will have heard, like poorly fitting trainers, increasing mileage too quickly, running on hard surfaces all the time, poor biomechanics and other assumptions. The fact is we are drawing parallels that may not be there. There is evidence to show that in most cases, it's just one leg that is affected; yet studies have shown the non-injured side also has the same pathology. I have read information recently suggesting there is a hormonal element or other centralized cause for the injury and more results from these studies may well develop this idea further in time.

The one thing that we know to be true is that we don't know everything yet. The methods used to treat an Achilles have changed more times since I became a physiotherapist than the approach to any other injury. Research is always evolving in this area and there are a greater number of research papers currently, largely owing to the increased numbers of those suffering. There is an audience hungry for this information and where there is need there will be development.

PROGRESSION OF THE INJURY

Research indicates that the injury is caused by the Achilles breaking down, that the collagen fibres start to spread and ground substance (water-based, gel-like substance found in connective tissue) infiltrates the spaces between them. With this expansion of the fibres comes an increase in Achilles size, usually in the distal 1/3 of the tendon, just above the heel. The tendon is usually 0.6cm from back to front and a thickened Achilles will increase towards a full centimetre. This can be measured using either ultrasound scan (USS) or magnetic resonance imaging (MRI). My preference is a USS as you can scan in real time, scan through movement and also switch to dopla mode to look for blood vessel involvement.

SELF-ASSESSMENT

If you have the feeling of stiffness and pain in your Achilles tendon in the morning when you first start to walk, then it's likely you have a tendon issue. Try first of all squeezing the tendon along its length and see if you identify a clearly defined 'most painful' spot. Take hold of the Achilles tendon with both fingertips and gently distort the tendon lifting with one hand and pulling with the other so it bends side to side. If this elicits pain, then, given nothing else is being manipulated, it's likely the issue does lie with the tendon itself.

Try a stretch to the tendon (a calf stretch off a step) and if this also gives some pain, you are likely to have an Achilles problem.

Most tendon issues outside of a rupture will ease after a period of activity, if only for a short time, but then the pain will come back if the exercise continues. Test this with a walk of about 15–20 minutes to see if the pain reduces significantly.

If your tendon is behaving as per above, then available physiotherapy is now very well researched and successful. Get in touch with a physiotherapist sooner rather than later.

TREATMENT

Achilles tendinopathy can be treated with several modalities from the physiotherapist, but there are also surgical options.

The physiotherapist will use soft tissue massage on the calf muscles and into the foot, ankle joint mobilizations and foot mobilizations. You may well be prescribed in-shoe orthotic inserts if the biomechanics of the foot and ankle are perceived to be at fault. Eccentric or appropriate loading as outlined in the next section are the key route to being free from this common running ailment.

However, if the appropriate loading process fails, for those resistant tendons that just don't respond to the normal physiotherapy, there is shockwave therapy (SWT), a series of shocks derived from lithotripsy, which in layman's terms is breaking up of hard substances.

A reminder of what SWT is and does, as described earlier: SWT stimulates the immune system and releases nucleic acids within the target cells, which are the pre-requisites for any tissue healing. In order for healing to take place this process must occur and with SWT the initial process involves mechanical pressure, which increases the cell permeability, increasing local circulation to the tissues and increasing metabolism. Secondly, it breaks up any calcium deposits through the pressure front producing hundreds of thousands of cavitational bubbles that expand and then collapse creating a secondary force breaking up the calcific deposits. Cells responsible for soft tissue and bone regeneration and healing are known as fibroblasts and osteoblasts. SWT has been shown to stimulate these cells and therefore promote healing. Finally SWT has a pain-reducing element to it, working on the brain's transmission of pain, first of all as a transient, short-lived pain reduction, however it is also being shown to work on the 'pain-gate', acting as a reset button for the perception of pain and therefore having potential long-term effects on pain reduction.

Recent scientific study into SWT resulted in 75% of patients reporting their Achilles pain free at their six-month follow-up and a further 14% with greater than 50% reduction in pain.

There is also the option of a high volume injection, known as a bolus, whereby saline is injected between the tendon fibres and the fat pad

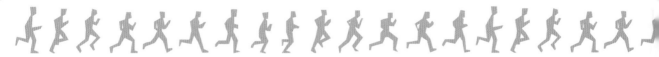

that sits anterior to it, thus separating the two (similar to a surgical intervention).

If you don't get better, there is a fairly new poly pill you can use under a GP's guidance. Recent research in sports science has indicated there's some evidence that putting three medications together actually has a beneficial effect on chronic tendon issues. Doxycycline (a penicillin available on prescription) taken 100mg per day, alongside 400mg of ibuprofen four times per day and as much green tea as you like; these three medications together make up the poly pill (Fallon, *et al.* 2008).

You are unable to self-administer this as you need a prescription from your GP for the Doxycycline, and just taking ibuprofen and green tea does not have the same effect at all, but may cause some stomach issues, so you absolutely have to discuss this with your GP before starting.

Finally, while I am not an advocate, there is always the option of surgery when it comes to the Achilles. Instead of looking to perform surgery on the Achilles itself, some orthopaedic surgeons favour cutting (resecting) the small muscle that sits alongside the Achilles 'plantaris' (however, not everyone has one to start with), as chronic Achilles pain can be attributed to an issue with the plantaris, and not the Achilles tendon itself. By having the plantaris surgically resected, some individuals have found their pain has subsequently gone. Following any surgery, there will be a period of rest that is then supported by a full rehabilitation plan of strength training, a part of all of these treatment options.

SELF-TREATMENT
The treatment centres around three key types of muscle contractions:

1 Isometric contraction
2 Eccentric contraction
3 Concentric contraction.

The key here is to understand how to do these contractions in the correct way at the correct time. Initially you may well be just matching resistance, contracting the muscle without movement known as isometric contraction. Then you can move onto eccentric exercises, whereby there is no load on the upward movement but resistance against the lowering back to the neural position. Finally concentric movements are included where by the muscle is being used in both the upward and lowering movements through range. The bicep muscle in the upper arm is an easier muscle to explain the movement patterns, for the patient to then take this model onto the more complex ankle movements.

The Achilles requires appropriate loading via exercise. 'Appropriate loading' means loading the tendon using the best methods for that individual to stress the fibres for optimal healing. It has always been universally accepted that eccentric loading of the Achilles through the heel raise (see page 179) is optimal for healing, however more recently there has been a move to heavy slow repetitions (HSR) (Bayer *et al*, 2015) whereby you use concentric and eccentric loading in a metronomic fashion, 3 seconds up and 3 seconds down. I have to say that I do still really like eccentric contractions, I have a lot of success with these over many years and whilst I always make sure they are performed with a heavy load (with a rucksack on your back for example) and performed slowly, I usually build a patients rehab to end with eccentric loading and you will see that throughout the book.

For any of these options, the patient may be in too much pain or lack the strength to perform any form of heel raise. In this instance an isometric contraction held for 45 seconds in mid range will not only start the strengthening process but may also reduce the pain levels. Heel raises, as in pushing up onto your toes, can be done in several different ways. The heel raise can be done from the flat surface up onto tiptoes, or lowering off a step, enabling a greater degree of movement into dorsiflexion. There are also single leg and double leg variations, as well as with the feet positioned for internal or external rotation. Such is the variety, it's difficult to give just one method of exercising all Achilles injuries, however, the norm would be as follows:

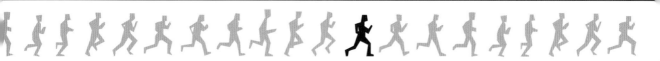

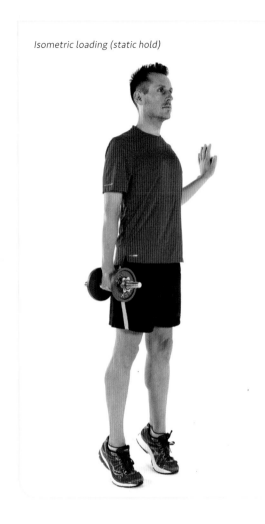

Isometric loading (static hold)

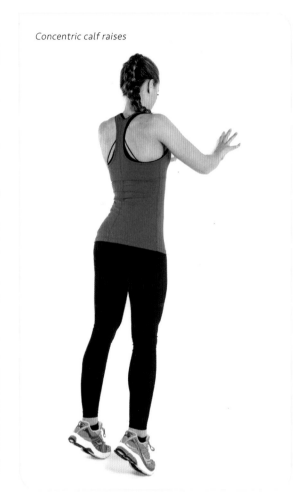

Concentric calf raises

Start with isometric loading (muscle contraction without movement), see above.

- Stand on the floor using the wall for balance if necessary. You can add weight through handheld dumbbells or a filled rucksack (to keep your hands free)
- Lift up onto your tiptoes and hold for 45 seconds
- Slowly lower down and return to the floor.

For isometric exercise, hold this pose for approximately 45 seconds at a time and repeat 4 times. As mentioned with the ankle previously, hold this pose with the heel different distances from the floor so as to gain strength through range.

Move to single leg isometric holds after a few days.

Perform concentric calf raises from the floor (moving onto tiptoes before lowering yourself down). Move to double leg then single leg as you are able to progress. Do 3 x 15 reps per day for 3 weeks.

Then move onto the eccentric calf raises (page 179). Eccentric loading is where you only stress the muscle on the return against gravity or resistance. Therefore you need to do as little work as possible to get into the start position on tiptoes, then work in a slow motion down to the end of your available ankle range (which has to be done single leg), 3 x 15 reps with weight on alternate days. Lower slowly, taking 6 seconds from tiptoes to end range, then raising up either with support or using the good leg back to the starting point.

The process of appropriate loading for the Achilles has an effect at the local cellular level and also builds strength. The cells become 'upset' by the excess load and respond with proteins to protect themselves.

WHAT TO EXPECT FROM A PHYSIOTHERAPIST

Your physiotherapist should take the time to explain the Achilles so you understand the stages of rehabilitation that are required. The weight of responsibility lies on your shoulders to ensure that you understand and are compliant with the home exercise programme (HEP) of appropriate loading. But in the interim, your physio will want to see you fortnightly for treatment and assessment. Expect your exercises to get harder every four weeks.

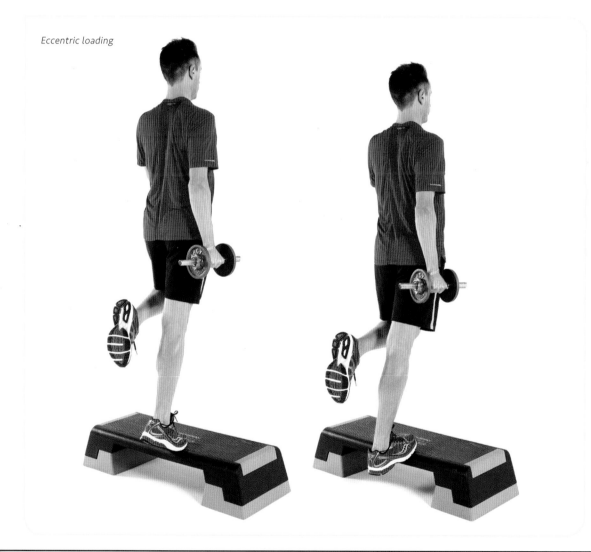

Eccentric loading

PRACTITIONER PROTOCOL

- Assess if this is mid-portion Achilles pain or insertional
- Provide advice on the nature of the injury and how it reacts to exercise so your patient fully understands the effects and benefits of the exercises prescribed
- The appropriate loading of the Achilles for your patient is very personalized. You need to perform a good assessment and decide what best suits their needs. If unsure then start with 45 second holds of isometric contractions x3, repeated 3 times per week, for a couple of weeks. Move onto HSR, 15 reps x3 on a 3 second up and 3 second down ratio. If relevant then move onto eccentric loading.

Most of all make sure your patient knows this is a long term exercise prescription that needs to be kept up for as long as they intent to keep running.

Treatments should be as follows, every other week, so 7 sessions in total, to include:

- SSTM to the gastrocnemius and soleus
- Ankle mobes and foot mechanics optimized through mobilization of tarsal joints
- DTF to the Achilles
- Shockwave therapy 4 applications 7 days apart, 500 shocks at 10 per second/1.5Htz, followed by 2000 shocks at 10 per second 2.5Htz.

Being pain-free during the protocol is not a reason to stop the exercises or to cease physiotherapy. See the whole 12-week process through to its conclusion if you want the best possible result.

GETTING BACK TO RUNNING

The thing I love about the Achilles is the ability to keep running when it's injured. The strapline for the Achilles tendon is 'push into pain', such is the ability of the structure to respond to a positive stress being applied. The Home Exercise Programme should be heavy and hard to complete, and as such the individual is able to continue to run, but with two essential caveats:

1 You can only run if the pain felt is lower than a 4/10 on the visual analogue scale (VAS).

2 The second caveat is that pain shouldn't increase either during a run or throughout the week. So this means that you can actually still be within caveat number 1 with a VAS of 2/10 but have to stop if it rises to a 3/10. You therefore need to pay attention to both rules independently and simultaneously.

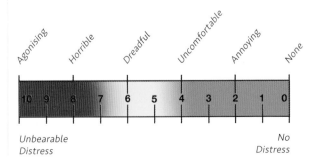

| Agonising | Horrible | Dreadful | Uncomfortable | Annoying | None |

10 9 8 7 6 5 4 3 2 1 0

Unbearable Distress   No Distress

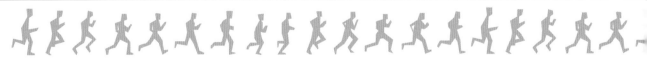

I was training for the London Marathon in 2009 and had put in lots of work in the hope of achieving my goal of completing the race in less than three hours, so in March, a month before the marathon, I ran a tune-up race in preparation. The race couldn't have gone any better, I felt strong and knocked four minutes off my previous personal best – I was in great shape and ready to achieve my goal.

The following day, however, I got out of bed and had a shooting pain through my Achilles tendon and lower calf muscle. I put this down to general stiffness and having tired muscles after the previous day's exertions. I fully expected the pain to subside as the day went on.

As the days and weeks went by the pain in my leg continued, the worst times being getting out of bed in the morning and walking down stairs, and as I had to try to train to keep the sub 3 dream alive, the first 10 minutes of each run.

I toyed with the idea of pulling out of the marathon but after all of the hours and miles I'd put into training I couldn't bring myself to do it.

Race day came around and I took my place on the start line full of pain killers, hoping that I could somehow race well after my final month's training had been virtually nonexistent. By 10 miles my running style had turned into a limp and I knew I wouldn't complete the race. At 13 miles I found an underground station that I could use to get back to the finish. Once I'd collected my kit from the finish area I sat in St James's Park and cried. On the train home from the race I vowed that I'd never be in that position again.

As I'd tried to continue to train and attempted to race on my injured Achilles, I later found that I'd torn the muscle. Because I'd made such a mess of it, it took me a full 18 months to be back running pain free.

By 2012 I was ready to give the marathon my all again and I began to prepare for the 2013 London Marathon. I committed fully to my training again still with the aim of completing the course in under three hours. In January 2013 I began to get the same Achilles pain in the mornings whilst going down the stairs that I'd had previously. This time though I didn't waste any time hoping the pain would just disappear and booked an appointment with Paul.

I ran on the treadmill so Paul could assess my running style, gait and foot plant, and from this he got a clear picture of what was going on. He then had me lay on the physio bed to see what muscle groups were tight or inflamed. Paul diagnosed the injury to be Achilles tendinopathy and Calcaneal bursitis.

From this assessment, he devised a stretching and strengthening routine for me, which included eccentric calf lowering exercises and weighted calf lowering exercises enabling me to quicken the recovery.

As I'd had physio early on, before it developed fully, I was able to complete pretty much all of the training I had planned.

Through continuation of the exercises prescribed and regular visits to Paul for friction rubs to promote blood flow, sports massage and completing more of my training runs on grass and avoiding hills where possible, my injury cleared up well before race day.

This time I took my place on the start line for the marathon feeling very confident. The whole day was fantastic with the sunny streets of London lined with thousands of people supporting us all and spurring us on, and to top it all off I had my family and nine-month-old daughter cheering me on in the final miles. I crossed the line in a time of 2:52:11. Finally I'd attained my goal, four years after I'd set out to achieve it. Obviously a large part of it was down to the training effort, but I certainly wouldn't have achieved it without the help, knowledge and support of a great physiotherapist.

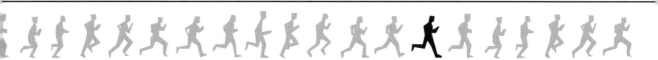

CHAPTER 3

THE LOWER LEG

There won't be a runner out there who hasn't at some point had a lower leg issue. The lower leg is the area with the most common running injuries after the knee. When you look at the biomechanics of the runner, be it forefoot or heel-toe techniques, you will see strain, rotation and ground reaction forces that have to be absorbed in the lower leg.

The injuries we will be focusing on here are:

- Shin splints
- Calf strains
- Peroneal tendinopathy
- Head of fibula pain
- Compartment syndrome
- Tibial stress fracture.

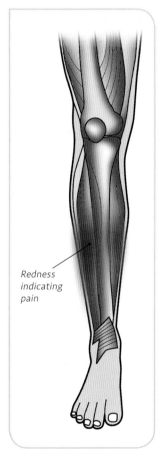

Redness indicating pain

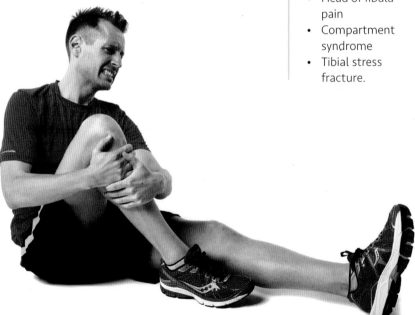

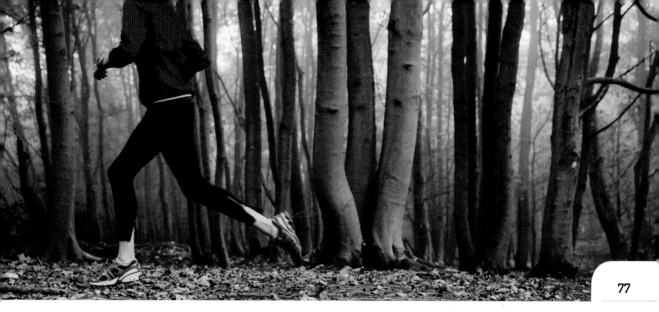

Shin splints

What is it?

'Shin splints' is the non-medical term for medial tibial stress syndrome (MTSS) (Czyzewski, 2012). Shin splints are the bugbear of so many runners, especially for those runners in their second month of training for their first marathon or half marathon. It's my experience that runners tend to get more injured in their first year of training than in the whole of the following five years!

EARLY WARNING SIGNS

- Tightening of the calf muscles in the few runs leading up to the shin pain
- Dull aching pain at the front of the lower leg – usually the medial ⅓ of the shin
- Pain usually at the start and then the end of the run initially
- As the injury progresses pain will get worse with every minute of running
- Pain will develop and be present even when walking
- Pain on lifting the toes against resistance
- Loss of ankle plantarflexion (pointing toes).

COMMON REASONS FOR INJURY

Risk factors have been shown to be increased body mass index (BMI), poor alignment of the small bones in the foot, a loss of plantarflexion (ability to point the toes) and a loss of hip rotation externally (Baker *et al.*, 2001). What this means is that there are key factors of a biomechanical nature that cause overload to the muscles of the lower leg. These muscles can be overloaded through poor biomechanics and also over-training, therefore to fully understand the mechanism of injury is the route to complete rehabilitation.

When you run, your foot is lowered under control by key lower leg muscles, which often become fatigued and stop being so effective. This is most common when training is stepped up too rigorously and too quickly. Muscles need a chance to develop in size, strength and flexibility, and most people who lift weights know not to do bicep curls every day, yet running is basically the same as working the equivalent muscle in the lower leg in this way. The muscle cannot sustain the constant lifting and slow lowering of the foot over continually increasing distances without adequate rest. When I set training programmes for beginners I am so careful to allow for these changes as well as bone density development, cardiovascular changes and the like. In fact, as

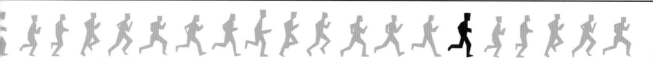

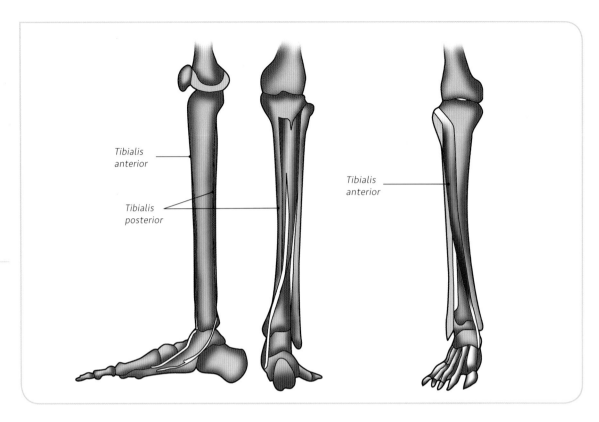

Tibialis
anterior

Tibialis
posterior

Tibialis
anterior

we move up to the knee and hip sections of this book, the significance of recovery for these areas and the potential risks of ignoring this advice will be revealed in all their horrible glory.

To help the tsunami of shin pain sufferers each year I have developed a package of treatment that seems to nip this one in the bud with impressive speed. The key is to provide strengthening exercises to the appropriate muscles, which make the injury-prone lower leg more robust, whilst strengthening and lengthening the muscle tissue and thereby correcting the common biomechanical faults.

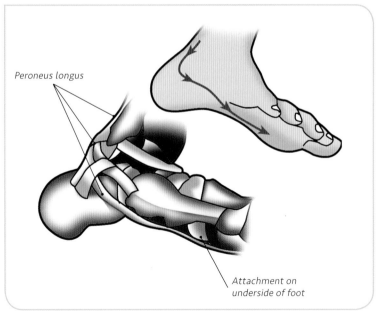

Peroneus longus

Attachment on
underside of foot

The muscles that are particularly overworked and stressed are tibialis posterior and tibialis anterior.

These muscles act like the reins of a horse, directing and determining the speed of travel for the foot. They work in conjunction with the peroneal longus and brevis muscles.

Both the peroneal longus and tibialis posterior attach under the foot and therefore provide this stabilizing role. These soft tissues become inflamed at their attachments to the outer layer of the bone known as the periosteum. There is pain associated with this inflammation and also the attachments/adhesions of the soft tissues to the bone.

PROGRESSION OF THE INJURY

If you continue to run, you will keep aggravating the periosteum causing more inflammation known as periostitis.

The muscle will not become stronger if you just try fighting through this pain. It will become worse and could lead to additional stress being placed through the bones of the shin and foot. The inability to lower the foot slowly enough or with enough control due to increasing muscle fatigue results in an overuse injury. The foot will begin to land noisily and without control, and the stress therefore will be driven up the leg and the potential for a stress fracture increased.

SELF–ASSESSMENT

Feel along your shin and see if there is a painful spot in the lower ⅓ of the shin towards the inside edge of the bone. If this pain is over an area of at least a few centimetres and up to the whole length of the lower half, then it is potentially shin splints. However, if the pain is very specific, between 1 and 15 millimetres, with little or no pain either side, then take a look at the section on tibial stress fracture on page 98 for reference.

A secondary assessment is to sit with your legs out straight with bare feet. Allow your feet to fall naturally, not pushed down. Assess the injured side versus the non-injured side and see if the foot is more upright, suggesting tighter muscle in the anterior shin. You may also see tension in the muscle tibialis posterior causing your foot to turn inwards as well.

TREATMENT

The treatment is threefold: 1) to stop further injury, 2) reduce inflammation and to strengthen, and 3) lengthen the muscle tissue. Therefore there is a period of 'relative rest', which means rest from the aggravating activity, but not just sitting on your couch for the next six weeks. There are plenty activities you can still do to keep fit and aid the rehabilitation. For the inflammation and healing promotion, use ice and compression, and for the muscle rehabilitation, the introduction

'PRONE' TO SIMPLIFY?

Now we are talking biomechanics, it's important to realize the role this element plays. People at high risk of this injury are those with poor biomechanics. For years 'over-pronation' was viewed as a cause of this shin pain. The foundation for this idea was that by supporting the rear foot and longitudinal arch, there was less pressure being placed on the tibialis posterior for foot control and less rotation of the tibia through the gait cycle. However this is a simplistic view and we need to assess the individual runner as far up as the hip and pelvis if we are to fully diagnose and rehabilitate.

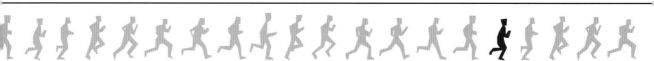

of a stretch and strengthening programme. There is also a need to look at the wider biomechanics to assess if there is an overload of the tibialis muscle group as result of poor form, or to exclude this and instead research the training load prior to injury for signs of overuse.

Calf tightening is very common and therefore we cannot ignore this as part of the treatment and rehabilitation. Soft tissue on the calf muscles should be the start point in the treatment process: to release any built-up tension. The physiotherapist will work to separate the muscles in order to get them working as their individual components. The blood flow increase brings with it an analgesic effect, therefore making this slightly more comfortable for you to cope with, given this is a deep and sometimes painful treatment. The soft tissue techniques work to break down any adhesions between the soft tissues and the bone, restoring optimal function. During this process the increased blood flow goes some way to releasing pain-reducing hormones

SELF-TREATMENT
From the exercise appendix choose exercises: Towel grabbing (strength), page 167, Calf (stretch), page 168, Soleus (stretch), page 168, Calf raises (strength), page 169, Toe raises (strength), page 169, Tibialis posterior (strength) page 170, Shin (stretch), page 171 and Glutes (stretch) page 177.

This is a large number of stretches, however if all are done in one session it will still take less than 20 minutes, which is less time than you would have spent running when not injured. You do need to see rehab as alternative to running in this instance and ring-fence the time you would have used running for your rehab.

WHAT TO EXPECT FROM A PHYSIOTHERAPIST
Physio for shin splints can be quite uncomfortable, as there is a need to release muscle tension and work quite deep and close to the tibia (shin bone). You will be given a lot of exercises to do away from physiotherapy (see above) and you may be

PRACTITIONER PROTOCOL

- SSTM to the gastrocnemius and soleus (these often tighten before the onset)
- Ankle mobilization and foot mobilization
- If after assessment it appears there is excessive rear foot pronation, a trick I use is to insert 4° rear foot varus wedges from www.canonbury.com (made by Vasyli Orthotics) attaching these to the trainer insole during rehabilitation to reduce this, which allows the tibialis posterior a reduced load
- Deep treatment to the anterior shin, between the bone and the soft tissues, three long lines up the inside edge to release any adhesions
- Despite the potential for bruising in this area, repeat this treatment weekly until pain-free
- Start back running once the pain is reduced to below 4/10 VAS and only for three-minute intervals at a steady pace on a treadmill incline (unless you have access to an alter-G treadmill, in which case you can start almost immediately).
- Build the patient back to running by reducing the rest periods and increasing the intervals.

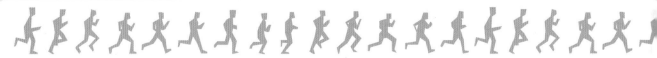

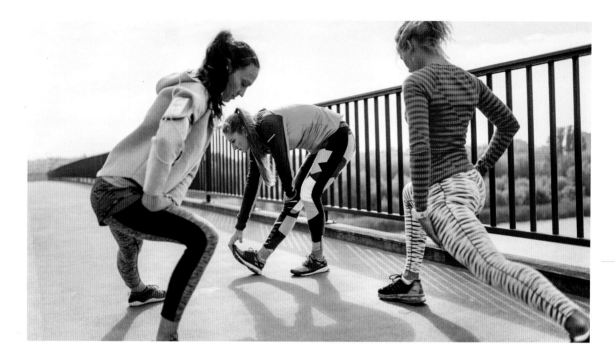

recommended an orthotic insole to reduce the stress within the foot and shin during walking/running.

GETTING BACK TO RUNNING

Interestingly, running on a treadmill with an incline (providing you have adequate flexibility to do so) can be effective at keeping impact and pain to a minimum and is more exercise-specific in terms of keeping a training programme going. Where possible you should try to move straight to this form of exercise, although in cases where there is pain on walking, you may need to resort to aqua jogging or cross training before hitting the treadmill.

Once you can do some work on the treadmill, it's important to pace this work. Often the temptation is to run until you feel pain, but it is imperative that instead you anticipate the potential pain and, through regular stops, keep the soft tissues long and free from tension. Stop after a short period of running and measure the reaction over the coming hours. In a great number of cases the calf muscle was the first thing to tighten, so stopping at regular intervals to stretch the calf during these

rehab runs not only maintains some length, but affords the tibialis posterior and associated muscles time to recover. My favourite session to start with is 5 x 3 minutes with the stretch stops, and this session is repeated throughout an array of injury rehab protocols in this book.

Slowly but surely, it is possible to extend these running intervals and increase the overall running time in small, calculated steps, for example 5 x 4 minutes, then 5 x 6 minutes. These rehab runs must work alongside the rehabilitation exercises that are strengthening and lengthening the muscle groups. It is vital that the strengthening exercises prescribed are not performed prior to running, or even in the few hours before going for a run. Strengthening exercises fatigue muscle and therefore increase the injury risk. The foolproof method is to do strength in the evening before bed and run during the first half of the day, though not straight from bed with tight, cold muscles.

Beware – the reason the treadmill incline works is because the forefoot doesn't have as far to travel, therefore reducing the workload on the

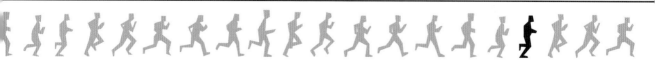

muscles involved. Therefore it's not right to simply lower the incline and continue along the same training duration and intensity – instead, as the incline comes down, so should the duration of your intervals. Not all the way back to the start point of 5 x 3 minutes, but certainly 30% less than you have been doing with the incline.

You then build back up in exactly the same way you did with the incline. This doesn't mean you have to run less distance each session, as you can add in periods of incline running as well to keep your training going forwards.

Then you have a transition to running outside again, gradually building this back into your routine, with periods of treadmill running in the same proportions as when reducing the treadmill incline.

Conversely to the treadmill incline reducing impact, running downhill increases it. When you

CLIENT STORY: CHRIS, 24

When I began doing athletics two years ago, I was training for the 800m. Training had been going well in the first year, however, no matter what I did, I couldn't seem to break the two-minute barrier. At the end of the season I joined another training group that was more specific to the 800m. We trained incredibly hard all winter and I was noticing massive gains in my endurance. However, in this group we drastically increased the mileage on the road. This in turn gave my shins a pounding and towards the end of the winter training, coming in to spring, I developed shin splints.

The best way to describe it is similar to a toothache-like pain in the shins and very tender to the touch. I had pain for around a month and it was gradually getting worse. It never felt too bad whilst actually running but the aching pain would begin after returning home after a session. I didn't know how to combat this, so continued to train through it until the pain became even worse.

I had been to Paul a number of times for sports massage, so I decided to visit him and get my shins seen too. Initially he assessed my full body comparing it to my last visit a number of months beforehand. He then began to massage my shins, which was ridiculously painful. I was given a number of drills and exercises to complete on a daily basis and was also told to wear cushioned trainers more and to ice my shins after every session.

He recommended having a week off running and to instead use the bike and do aqua jogging. This I felt would be a big issue as I had worked so hard over the winter and the season was about to start. I was advised not to wear lightweights/spikes on the track – and again I felt bad about this as the rest of my group was doing fast track sessions in lightweights or spikes. I also had to cut down on my long Sunday run and instead do 90 minutes on the bike. I was sticking to all of the advice but didn't feel happy at all because the season was starting.

After around eight weeks of regular physio visits, doing the exercises and rehab for my shins, I could finally feel the aching feeling becoming less and less after each session. I then gradually got back into my Sunday runs, starting at 3 miles building back up to 10 over a number of weeks. I kept to wearing my cushioned trainers on the track for another six weeks and then got into the racing flats for faster sessions, which felt great. The next time I wore spikes was in a race, and I broke the two-minute barrier with 1.57.

I was amazed that after feeling so down not being able to train properly for almost three months I managed to get a PB at the end of that season. I stuck with my regular physio visits and rehab thoughout all of that season and think that if I hadn't got physio, I would have ended up only getting worse problems with my shins, which could have led to more severe problems.

start to run outside again, you have to be extremely careful how you tackle the downhill sections of your run. It's fine to run short and slow sections of downhill, but not all of us live on Salisbury Plain or the pancake that is Florida, in fact where I live in Northumberland, you are either running up a hill or down one. It's so important that you start to think about not just how you are doing your rehab but where, and in what conditions.

Calf strains

What is it?

We've all had that agonizing moment when the pull in our calf is beyond that of a mere muscle contraction and within seconds we have had to stop running. Or the feeling that someone just shot us in the back of the leg and the need to pull up is immediate. Rarely, due to the nature of the calf's role in running, is it possible to run through a calf issue. This muscle group is so integral to our propulsive force, it's the mainstay of our balance, and it operates the mechanics of the foot and assists the hamstrings in their role (Campbell, 2009). Unfortunately, there isn't an additional muscle to rely on or any technique that allows you to keep going, so there's no way to keep on running.

EARLY WARNING SIGNS
- Sudden onset of acute pain whilst out running
- Calf tightens immediately
- Pain level is often quite severe
- Unable to load through the foot normally causing a limp
- Pain is increased with loading.

COMMON REASONS FOR INJURY
So what happens when a calf muscle injury hits? The medial gastrocnemius is believed to have over 1.2 million muscle fibres, therefore if the lateral gastrocnemius had a similar amount and the soleus were to have around 800,000, then the calf complex

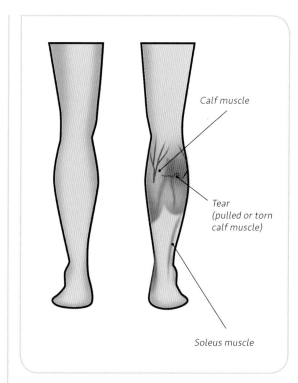

Calf muscle

Tear (pulled or torn calf muscle)

Soleus muscle

would have over 3 million available muscle fibres per leg (Feinstein *et al.,* 1955).

During an injury, some of the fibres of the muscle cell over-stretch and tear. Muscle fibres are something that have to either be switched on or off, like a light switch. There is no middle ground, we modulate muscle fibre recruitment based upon the perceived muscle force required to perform certain tasks. In the case of running, a mere few hundred thousand muscle fibres might be needed for each stride, but these fibres fatigue as their turn to fire up again comes round again and again. It's usually just as you start up a hill well into your run that the calf grabs and starts to hurt. On the flat, your fibres were sharing the workload of pushing your body up and forwards with timetabled accuracy. When you met the hill, the assumption by your brain was that to get up the hill, more fibres would be required for each step, but the rapid and increased recruitment meant the fibres were caught napping and being already fatigued, some buckled under the strain.

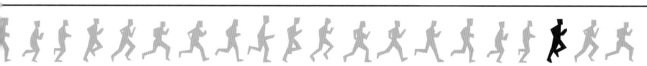

PROGRESSION OF THE INJURY

A calf tear usually causes you to stop running immediately; in fact you will have little say in the matter, as to run on will be impossible due to the pain and loss of strength. Therefore there is in effect no progression of this injury except if you decide to return to running too quickly afterwards.

It is alarmingly common for someone to pull a calf muscle quite badly but feel capable of running again after three weeks of rest and then pull it again on the second time they try to jog. Why is this? This is due to how muscle fibres operate, as discussed before: when walking the recruitment is fairly low, so after a short period of the healing process there is no pain on walking. In fact, many people can produce some pretty impressive single leg calf raises and be convinced that going for a slow run will be OK. Largely speaking it is, but the second time you go out, it might be just that little bit faster, with therefore a greater recruitment of fibres and faster turnaround of use between the fibres within the unit. A slight incline or even a push up to return to a path from the road will be enough to increase the tear and take with it any immature fibres from the healing process.

SELF-ASSESSMENT

The ability to identify this is difficult at times for a physiotherapist, so self-assessment is tricky to say the least. However, proceed with caution and get some cooking oil on your fingertips and start to rub this in over the whole muscle, gradually get deeper and deeper, looking for the most painful spot. See if your fingertips appear to dip in at the most painful spot, or if the surface of the muscle is smooth and just sensitive. Sometimes, you can feel an actual dip in the muscle, suggestive of a slight tear.

See if the strength is reduced, but don't overload an injured muscle too much. Sit with your feet against a wall or door and push against it. You will feel pain and weakness in the calf that is affected. Damaged muscle will be weak and painful, use this as your guide, but the overriding point to be made here is that it is tough for you to self-assess, so seek a local physiotherapist trained to do so.

TREATMENT

In the event of this injury occurring, you must stop immediately. Most of the time you will want to anyway or rather be unable to continue. With an injury to a muscle such as this, it has always been thought that you rest, apply ice initially and some form of compression. As previously discussed, the use of ice is in debate at this stage of injury. I do not advocate you using any form of ibuprofen however, as it interferes with the immediate healing response elicited from the body's natural defences. You must delay any non-steroidal anti-inflammatory drug (NSAID) for three to four days to allow for the collagen synthesis to take place.

Initially after the injury there is an acute inflammatory phase lasting up to four days as the body prepares for repair. The repair phase peaks at three weeks, with the remodeling phase continuing over months. Within the first 12 hours there are signs of early capillaries (tiny blood vessels) that will develop over the next few days. This is the period of redness, heat, swelling and pain. There are significant vascular and cellular changes taking place during this initial period which historically were left to R.I.C.E., the aim of this early management to reduce heat and swelling and promote healing and for new healthy tissue to have the optimum chance of development. There are some studies that suggest the body should be left to manage this phase on its own (Malanga et al., 2015; Tiidus, 2015). In the absence of any new findings, I think it is safest to continue using ice on acute tissue injury and to keep treating with rest, ice, compression and elevation.

There are some significant benefits to physiotherapy despite all these restrictions, which in most cases means gentle mobilizations, such as to the ankle joints to ensure that these continue to move optimally despite their reduced use throughout the period of injury. There is a great deal of benefit to simply being shown what you can and cannot do, plus being shown ways to apply strapping.

Compression is a buzzword at the time of writing (Hill et al., 2014) and the calf is an area

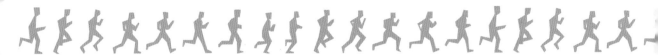

where people have found anecdotal benefit both as a training aid and as a rehabilitation aid, but the scientific community remains unconvinced beyond perceived benefit. I would suggest using a good quality calf guard during the immediate management of a calf tear.

Work hard to contain the swelling through applying compression and ensure that you rest the muscle as much as possible. As the pain and swelling subside and it becomes easier to walk once more, then it is time to think pragmatically about the route back to running. The usual time period to this point is six weeks from initial injury. Physiotherapy has a raft of treatment options for you throughout the stages of repair. Initially diagnosis, early management and some gentle but effective treatment options in clinic can be followed up through the stages of healing to become more rigorous and targeted to ensure that you optimize healing times, and most importantly that the muscle is repairing in the best way possible to prevent future injury.

Your physiotherapist can work on the muscle more and more as the repair process continues and will ultimately be in a position to provide a graduated return to training. In the early stages, rest is paramount, but as the repair process develops, treatments will ensure that scar tissue does not affect the future ability of the muscle, that the length and breadth of the muscle is maintained. Strengthening and stretching work must be carried out in the right proportions and using the correct technique throughout the process. Just reading a Google post on stretching a calf muscle doesn't mean that it's the right thing to do in the early stages. In fact, stretching should only be done once the muscle can provide pain-free resistance.

So you can see that it is not as simple as following a 1, 2, 3 approach. Physiotherapy guidance is incredibly important right from the outset, but do not become underwhelmed by the lack of deep manual work initially – there is plenty of time for this, but only once you have achieved some key milestones, dependent upon the severity of the injury.

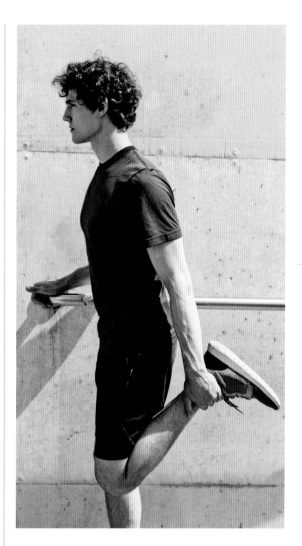

SELF-TREATMENT

Aqua jogging, cross training and if available an antigravity treadmill are all great ways to keep your running training going without causing more injury.

It is important to allow the soft tissues time to heal and to be compliant with the treatment schedule and advice of your physiotherapist. Sometimes the best treatment is rest and in the case of the calf muscle, feeling OK to walk is not a good measure of your ability to start to run. The soft tissues take six weeks to repair and then the road to recovery starts.

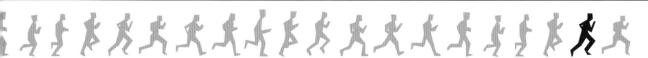

PRACTITIONER PROTOCOL

- Explanation of the muscle fibre recruitment goes a long way here, explaining that fibres contract either 100% or not at all and it's the number of fibres used that generates the force. This way, patients can understand why they can seemingly walk pain-free but then try to run and end up injured again and again
- The tension within the muscle can increase and yet stretching is potentially damaging to the immature repair, so soft tissue massage can be very useful in the early stages
- Kinesiology tape can't help with muscle repair. However, it can support the ankle joint and I have used this to great advantage whilst the calf muscle is recovering
- Eccentric calf raises, with zero concentric load to begin with, 3 x 15 on alternate days, no added weight
- With short rehab runs on a pain-free calf muscle I have managed to get patients started on some running specific rehab from four weeks post injury, but perhaps to stay on the safe side start at six weeks
- Compression guards for the calf appear to have a significant benefit during the return to play period of rehab, if nothing more than compression over the site, I do think there is a protective and venus return element that is useful and so I ensure all patients are advised of their use.

Perform these exercises: Calf (stretch), page 168, Soleus (stretch), page 168, Calf raises (strength), page 169, Tibialis posterior (strength), page 170 and Single leg balance, page 171.

WHAT TO EXPECT FROM A PHYSIOTHERAPIST
Typically a physiotherapist would only start working on the site of injury after 72 hours has passed, with some deep transverse frictions (DTF) for two minutes and six deep sweeps at the end as per the protocol for an acute injury. Deep transverse frictions are a form of manual therapy that aims to stimulate the cells to repair the soft tissue. Once the injury becomes chronic then they would look to do these DTF for 10 minutes. This type of treatment is not very painful once the initial soreness wears off from the numbing two-minute phase.

Expect some work around the ankle joints to ensure there is optimum movement and from a holistic approach the physio should look at tension in the hamstrings, hip flexors and even the thoracic spine, to make sure that poor posture had not been overloading the calf muscles as you run, creating an exaggerated forward flexion of the upper body and loading your centre of mass anteriorly.

Lastly, by providing some progressive strength and conditioning exercises to make your muscle unit more robust, they can help you reduce some of the negative influences of posture and running technique simply by having a stronger, more resilient muscle.

GETTING BACK TO RUNNING
Wait six weeks! Soft tissues need this amount of time to reproduce new tissue and become sufficiently robust to attempt more challenging

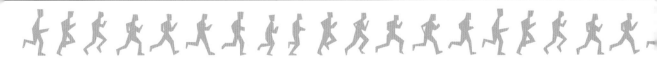

work such as running. Your rehabilitation exercises are designed to build this strength and resilience. Together these exercises (when combined with rest) will prepare you for the start of the return to running. Be patient and remember that despite your commitment to the rehabilitation exercises and diligently accessing physiotherapy, this is a muscle that has to work through its whole range of movement and is likely to injure again if stressed too early within the rehabilitation process.

CLIENT STORY: LAWRENCE, 44

I've been running since 1997, when a casual dare resulted in me running my first London Marathon the year after. After that first marathon, I was hooked and ran another six marathons and umpteen half marathons and 10k races over the next decade.

When I turned 40, for whatever reason, I decided to shake things up and put my trusted Asics 2040 shoes that had served me well aside and replaced them with Vibram FiveFinger shoes. Not only that, but I decided to try these new, glove-shaped shoes at the start of a two-month trip to Australia.

They were a bit weird at first, but after a week, I was hooked. I loved how light they felt which had the impact of me running faster and in what felt like a more natural way. I read books like Born to Run *and leapt into the world of barefoot running, filtering out the warnings that advised me to take it slow; and that maybe people with my background weren't designed to run barefooted! No. I knew best and wore my five finger shoes every day!*

Well, I kept running despite the pain in my left knee that appeared after a week. My instinct told me that something wasn't quite right, but as someone who likes to run every day, I ignored it, and hoped it would go away. Then the day before I returned to the UK, I got a terrible pain at the back of my calf. It was a terrible sharp pain that meant that I had to limp back to my hotel.

When I got back to the UK, I went to see Paul at Physio&Therapy who diagnosed a split in my calf muscle possibly as a consequence of my ongoing knee problem, a result of not giving myself time to adjust to a very different type of footwear!

Of course, none of this was a surprise and I just wanted the problem to be fixed that day! However, I was sent away taped up with blue tape and given a series of exercises to do daily, and advised NOT TO RUN FOR A WHOLE WEEK. This was tough to hear as in the 13 years that I'd been running, I'd only missed a couple of days!

I of course followed the approach and actually got into doing other types of exercises during that week, but was delighted when I was able to run again the following week. At this point, a sensible person would have stopped running barefooted. However, by this point, I was so used to running in the Vibrams and though I tried going back to Asics, in comparison they felt like concrete blocks! So I continued running in my Vibrams for the next four years.

During those four years, I had a range of similar problems, but then disaster struck while I was in Hong Kong; I got a terrible pain at the top of my foot that turned out to be a stress fracture. This was the final straw. Enough was enough. I hung up my FiveFinger shoes, returned to the 'concrete blocks', until eventually I settled on some great racing shoes that are more suitable and give me much more support.

However, good things always do come out of bad and the whole FiveFingers episode taught me that prevention is much better than cure. Whilst I learnt the hard way, I now stretch religiously every day and incorporate maintenance into my month to make sure that I am looking after my muscles so that they can continue to serve me well for a long time to come.

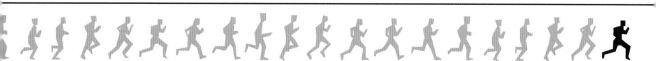

The general rules are to rest from running for six weeks, but work hard at your rehabilitation exercises, then at six weeks, focus on a steady return to your old running programme, taking time to stretch and strengthen between runs. Those who choose to simply rest passively for six weeks, then start back where they left off, will undoubtedly find themselves injured once more within the first two weeks.

Peroneal tendinopathy

What is it?

The peroneal muscle group is key in the lower leg. Think of them as one side of the 'reins' of the foot, the other side being the tibialis posterior (see the section on shin splints on page 77). This muscle group (made up of peroneus longus, tertius and peroneus brevis) works together to provide eversion (twisting the foot to the side – little toe first), and, in the case of longus and brevis, produce plantar flexion (pushing the foot down), whereas peroneus tertius provides dorsiflexion (lifting the foot upward).

EARLY WARNING SIGNS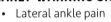

- Lateral ankle pain
- Pain like a tight band running down the lateral calf to the ankle and around the ankle bone
- Pain on toe off when walking
- Pain on eversion of the foot.

COMMON REASONS FOR INJURY

When you sprain an ankle the peroneal muscle can also become injured (Hertel, 2000) and will cause pain on contraction of the muscle. Of course in many cases both the ligaments and muscle are injured during an ankle sprain so the rehab is directed towards both. The peroneal muscle and tendon also become chronically injured through overuse, either as a result of inappropriately large increments in your training volume or through a biomechanical issue.

The two common ways to injury – muscle and tendon breakdown through overuse or an acute ankle sprain – will require different early management strategies. Acute sprains require approximately three days of natural healing, e.g. no intervention such as massage but the application of ice and strapping or support is very helpful, and without the use of NSAIDS (see page 12). Once out of the initial three days post-acute injury, however, the rehab aligns more closely with that of a chronic injury.

PROGRESSION OF THE INJURY

The injury to the peroneal muscle group is more often than not a tendinopathy, e.g. a problem with the tendon. This is due to injury or overload to the tendon. Research has shown that the inflammation period for a chronically injured tendon is short-lived or nonexistent, so referring to the injury as an inflammatory condition (tendonitis) is incorrect. Tendinopathy is the umbrella term for tendon disease, which is subdivided into either tendinosis – the chronic breakdown of the tendon where damage

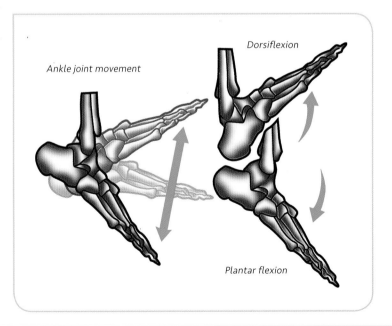

Ankle joint movement

Dorsiflexion

Plantar flexion

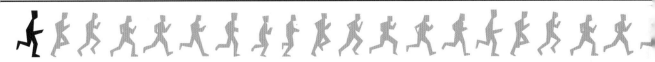

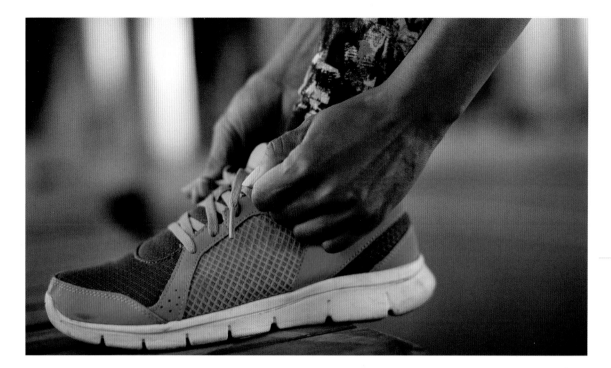

is at a cellular level – or tendonitis, which is acute damage and therefore does have inflammation, hence the accurate use of the suffix '-itis' for inflammation.

SELF-ASSESSMENT

Often following recovery from a sprained ankle, or a longer run, or with new shoes, you may notice pain on the lateral aspect of the ankle bone, possibly moving under the outside of your foot.

Test by resisting against pushing your foot down, also by rotating your ankle out to the side and then a combination of both. Just resist the movement with your hands and see if you get any pain in the same area. You are basically asking the muscle to work in the planes of movement it controls. Therefore, pain on resisted movement stresses the tendon and reproduces the same pain you are feeling.

Don't become confused with an ankle sprain and similar injuries to the area, like other tendon issues. The pain can subside with activity, only to return if the activity continues or following a period of rest.

TREATMENT

The treatment centres around three key types of muscle contractions:

1 Isometric contraction
2 Eccentric contraction
3 Concentric contraction.

We have discussed isometric, concentric and eccentric muscle action earlier (see page 71). These contractions can be performed through the three key ankle movements:

1 Eversion
2 Dorsiflexion
3 Plantar flexion.

The exercises that are most relevant in the early stages of rehab use isometric contraction owing to its low risk and because the exercise is able to develop quite quickly. Initially you will be instructed to hold your joint at a set position for

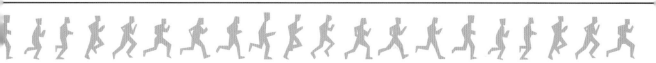

30–40 seconds, usually the mid-range of available movement. The development is then to produce the same duration hold at a variety of different joint angles, to develop this isometric strength through the available joint range. When doing an isometric exercise such as this, there are significant strength benefits, however the strength is gained at that particular joint angle and maybe 10 degrees either side. It is therefore necessary for you to hold the contraction at 30-degree intervals for the set period of time to ensure the joint has strength through its full range.

When performing this rehab on your ankle, there are many joint movements available. In order to better instruct you on how to perform isometric exercises for the peroneal muscles (commonly injured by an ankle sprain) let's first ensure we can achieve the necessary movements about the ankle.

Exercise: sitting in a chair with your legs outstretched before you, heels on the floor, see if you can evert the foot; that is, move the foot out to the side, not like a windscreen wiper but just so you show slightly more of the sole of your foot to someone sitting to your side.

Now try inversion, you will notice more available movement. Most people struggle with eversion and because of the pull of the muscles being used,

their foot tends to swing out to the side as well. You need to control this movement and just employ pure inversion and pure eversion. Take your time to correct yourself and experiment with both feet doing the same movement at the same time and then just using one foot.

Once you have mastered both inversion and eversion, now try to go through the three different muscle contractions against a resistance band. Producing the movement is relatively easy now, but see if you can perform pure eccentric contractions.

To do this you will need to release the tension from the exercise band, move the foot into eversion, then apply the tension without the foot moving. Once applied, slowly return the foot to neutral and then slightly beyond into inversion. Then release the tension fully, return the foot into the everted position and repeated the process.

SELF-TREATMENT

From the exercise appendix choose exercises Soleus (stretch), page 168, Calf raises (strength), page 169, Toe raises (strength), page 169, Tibialis posterior (strength), page 170, Peroneals–ankle eversion (strength), page 170 and Single leg balance page 171. These exercises should be done with an isometric (static) hold at first.

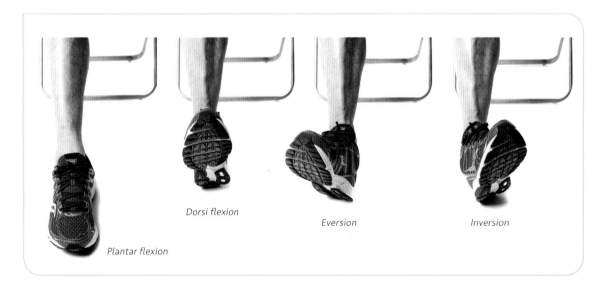

Plantar flexion

Dorsi flexion

Eversion

Inversion

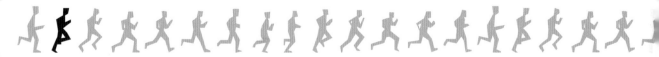

PRACTITIONER PROTOCOL

- SSTM to lateral lower leg, include soleus as well as peroneal longus muscle tissue
- DTF to the site of pain, on a stretch due to the shared peroneal sheath, so make sure you do these over a stretch
- The use of Shockwave therapy is very beneficial here, 500 shocks with 10 every second at 1.5Htz, then 2000 at 2.5 Htz
- Kinesiology tape is excellent to assist with recovery, taping to offload the lateral ankle. I would tape for several weeks until back running normal distances
- Depending upon the nature of the injury, a full gait analysis will be relevant only once the person is able to achieve 70% of their prior training programme so to have reduced any chance of antalgic gait or reduced muscle activity
- Eccentric eversion exercises from point of injury through until a month after full training has resumed.

Once you have mastered isometric contractions, you can move onto concentric contractions. A concentric contraction is where the muscle is moving into resistance and then the return movement is eccentric. Unless you have been told to do purely eccentric contractions then you will push or pull into the resistance for 15 repetitions, repeated 3 times per day. The number of these repetitions depends upon your athletic ability – some top athletes are capable of hundreds per day. Please be careful to moderate your repetition of these exercises according to your ability. In almost all cases, less is more in the early phase, but rehab becomes more aggressive as you approach a return to your running kit.

Eccentric exercise is the main one I would prescribe in the early stages of recovery from a tendon issue. Eccentric exercise is focusing purely on the return phase of the exercise. In the example of the plantar flexion exercise where you are pushing your foot down into the exercise band, the eccentric part is when you slowly return to the top with your foot closest to your shin. To perform a purely eccentric exercise, do not pull the resistance band at first and allow gravity to take your foot down into plantar flexion. Then hold it there whilst you pull on the band and create tension in an upward force. You can then resist the forces of the upward pull – slowly and in a controlled manner, allow your foot to come up into dorsiflexion, battling the resistance all the time. Release the band's tension at the end of that movement and start again. Three sets of 15 repetitions is again a set 'dosing' that works for most.

WHAT TO EXPECT FROM A PHYSIOTHERAPIST

The physiotherapist will want to identify which structure is at fault. The best way to do this on assessment is to go through a series of tests starting with passive movements whereby you do absolutely nothing and allow the physio to move your foot in all the end ranges of ankle and foot movement. The physio will be trying to recreate your 'pain', that is, the pain you feel sufficiently to present for physio. Other pains may come about as part of the testing which you need to identify as something else, perhaps just the pressure over a bruise on your toe. It is important for you to be specific about your pain, tell them as much as

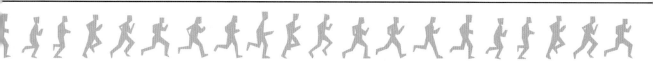

possible, grading the severity of pain between 0–10 where 10 is the most pain you can imagine and zero is no pain at all.

The physio will then get you to do all the same movements, using muscle contraction and finally ask you to resist those movements either in a static manner or through range. What this testing provides is an in-depth look at what structures are at fault, joint, ligament or muscle, each stressed differently by each test.

Depending upon how you sustained the injury you will then receive some treatment along the lines of manual therapy to the structure at fault and perhaps some kinesiology taping, but definitely the exercises described above.

GETTING BACK TO RUNNING

Peroneal tendinopathy and muscle strain can take as long as a calf strain or injured Achilles tendon before getting back to full training. However, I have seen clients return extremely quickly when the injury is identified early and treated appropriately. Unlike the calf strain or Achilles injury, the peroneal muscles respond well to taping (Jansen and Kamper, 2013) and this can accelerate the return to training with excellent results.

CLIENT STORY: BRENDON, 38

It was after a long ride that I noticed pain in the side of my leg. I was training for a half ironman distance at the time and combining a hard workload amongst swimming, cycling and running. As a triathlete you tend to get much less by way of injury when swimming or cycling and therefore running is always a concern, however, you have to train to be able to complete a half marathon on its own, let alone after an open water swim and long bike ride.

I know now that cycling wasn't the cause of my lower leg pain. After being assessed thoroughly from foot to hip by Paul, I was told my lateral calf muscles were tight due to the way I ran. Paul explained that I have high foot arches and he could see from the way that I ran on his treadmill that my feet tend to land heavily on the outside of my forefoot. This apparently has a shortening effect on my lateral calf muscles, placing a strain on the joint of the little lower leg bone called the tibia and the muscles that attach to it. Peroneal longus is the muscle that sits on the outside of the lower leg and Paul identified this as the main issue for me, including its nerve supply, which was becoming trapped.

I was interested in learning about my biomechanics and also that the problem I felt seemed to be as a result of an issue higher up in the leg than where I was feeling the pain. Having identified the cause of the pain, he was able to put me into some positions or ask me to do some tests that brought on the pain immediately. Paul then manipulated my leg (quite painful) just to the outside of my knee and I then repeated the tests – but with less than half the pain.

The rest of the session was largely unpleasant and I recall thinking 'no pain, no gain' but the after-effects were incredible. Within days I was back training, though not totally pain-free, but within two weeks I was totally free from pain. I continued with my exercises but Paul felt he had done enough treatment. I was shown a method of taping my ankle for some support and I repeated this for about four weeks. I was able to compete in all my triathlons that year, including the half ironman, which I completed in 5hr 39m.

I know when to see Paul; and the difference between a slight niggle and a possible problem. I now make sure that I do not fall foul of making a small injury worse and losing training time or not competing. With Paul's help and pragmatic advice and self-help treatments, I have been injury-free for more than a year.

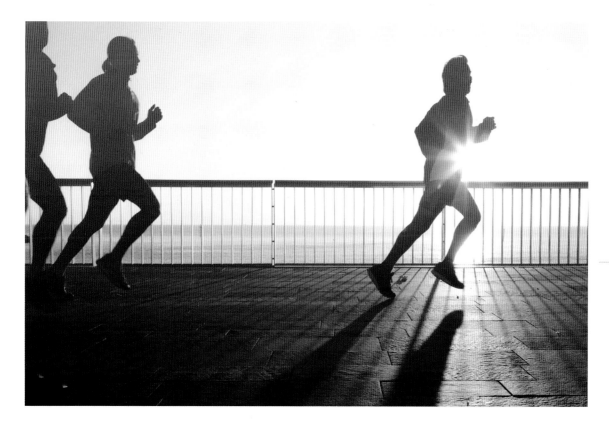

Head of fibula pain

What is it?

The head of the fibula is the small bony lump you can feel just lower than your lateral knee joint. It is the start of the smaller of the two lower leg bones (fibula) and is a non-weight bearing bone that articulates with the tibia, the larger of the two bones in the lower leg and the prime load bearer. Together, the fibula and tibia make up the first of the two ankle joints when they articulate with the talus bone in the foot (talocrural or mortise joint).

The interesting anatomy of the head of fibula is twofold. Firstly, the articulation with the tibia forms a small joint with fairly low significance, however, when this joint loses its minute amount of movement it can lead to pain at the site and lower down the lateral aspect of the leg. This is due to the second interesting part of the anatomy, which is the presence of the peroneal nerve, a primary branch of the sciatic nerve as it enters the lower leg. The nerve navigates around the head of the fibula and can become slightly impinged (Ryan *et al.,* 2003) at the site of the small tib/fib joint. The resultant and unwanted connection between the head of the fibula and the peroneal nerve causes nerve pain along the peroneal muscle group and into the lateral lower leg, ankle and even foot. Often misdiagnosed as an ankle sprain, peroneal tear or foot issue, it is a site that requires investigation and can be diagnosed using neural tension testing.

EARLY WARNING SIGNS
- Pain just below the knee on the lateral aspect of the lower leg
- Pain radiating along the lateral aspect of the lower leg down to the ankle and foot

- Burning or numbness or even pins and needles along the same distribution
- Numbness, pins and needles in the lateral foot.

Neural tension testing is a physiotherapy test whereby the nerves are put under gradual tension by adding certain physiological movements in turn, until the symptoms are felt (or not). You can attempt this test on your own: simply sit on a chair, totally relax your back so you 'slump' rather than bend forwards (I often tell clients to try and get your chin into your belly button as this generates the correct movement despite being pretty much impossible), then once in that position, start to straighten your injured leg. The test is positive if you feel your pain come on more and more as the leg straightens.

COMMON REASONS FOR INJURY
Often as a result of long runs in old trainers, poorly fitted shoes or poor biomechanics coupled with a rapid increase in training.

This issue can also come about following an ankle sprain, which goes relatively unnoticed until all the ankle pain and swelling has settled down and this is what you are left with.

PROGRESSION OF THE INJURY
If left without treatment, this injury can leave you with a constant burning sensation or that of a pulled muscle or strained ligament. The sensation itself (pins and needles or numbness) will increase over time and start to spread to a larger area.

SELF-ASSESSMENT
First, find your head of fibula by working your fingertips down from the outside of your knee past the knee joint line until you find an easily defined lump of bone. Beyond this lump you should be able to feel a continuous bone shaft, which should indicate you're in the right spot.

Take this bony lump (the head of fibula) between your thumb and forefinger and try to wiggle it side to side. It won't move but the action may be painful. If not, then try a little harder pushing it one way and then the next with more force using just the thumb. If either test produces more pain than the non-injured side, then the diagnosis is positive.

Now sit on a high chair or table top and floss your injured side as per Sciatic nerve flossing, page 180 in appendix 1. If this is more painful than your uninjured side, seek assistance from a physiotherapist.

PRACTITIONER PROTOCOL

- Soft tissue to the peroneal group, lateral calf group
- Ankle mobilizations
- Head of fibular mobilisations
- Provide exercises for nerve flossing (page 180) and calf stretches (pages 168 and 179)
- Repeat treatments for two weeks and see if pain has reduced sufficiently to resume running
- Check patient's trainers to see if there has been any collapse laterally
- Assess gait
- If trainers and gait are normal, assess the piriformis and pelvis for clues unless the injury arose from an acute ankle sprain or similar.

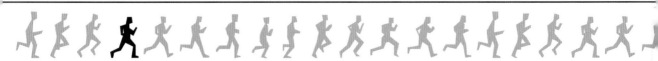

TREATMENT

The head of the fibula can be mobilized, thus restoring normal movement. This is done using manual therapy by a qualified practitioner. After some dedicated treatment, the neural tension testing can be performed again and differences noted. I have found this injury is really quite quick to resolve. If the mobilizations have worked successfully then I would prescribe something called nerve flossing to help keep the peroneal and sciatic nerves moving with their newfound freedom.

SELF-TREATMENT

Sciatic nerve flossing, page 180. Nerve flossing is a fairly underwhelming exercise when you are used to running or strength and conditioning training, as you feel very little. Essentially, you are sliding the tiny little nerves along their pathway from brain to foot, thus sliding the nerve past the head of the fibula each repetition maintaining the freedom of movement.

WHAT TO EXPECT FROM A PHYSIOTHERAPIST

The goal with this type of injury is to determine if this is a nerve entrapment issue or an actual soft tissue injury. If the soft tissue injury route is exhausted and the testing of neural tension is positive, then you may be surprised to have areas other than your pain spots worked on. This can be disconcerting as though the physio has missed the point. It's often alarming for someone to be working on the outside of your knee when the pain is in your big toe. Just wait for the results and have faith that the testing has been robust and the diagnosis accurate.

GETTING BACK TO RUNNING

Incredibly quick if the treatment is successful and in any case, this is a nerve issue and shouldn't detract from your ability to move, it may just be painful until you can get the area mobile once more.

CLIENT STORY: SUE, 28

I am at best a casual runner, not an athlete as such, but someone who enjoys exercising fairly regularly and is never more committed than when something is stopping me from running such as an injury. (We always want what we can't have).

One such time had not only me but several health care professionals perplexed, which was a pain along the outside of my left leg. One physiotherapist thought it was my knee, another thought compartment syndrome and yet no treatment seemed to make any difference.

It was a referral from a friend to see Paul at Physio&Therapy UK that made an instant difference. I explained the issue in about 4 minutes and before any testing or the pulling around of my leg as I had come to expect, I was told I had an issue with the little bone in my shin, or at least the joint at the top of that bone. I didn't believe it,

but one test was able to bring about all my pain immediately and yet seemingly take it away with a simple adjustment of the test, I couldn't believe it, this was a eureka moment for sure.

With a tiny amount of treatment the pain was gone, I don't mean a little bit gone I mean totally gone, albeit for a few hours, but it was the first time I felt I had found the cause of the problem. Three treatments later and I was back running pain free. I think the key to injury success is finding the right person to treat the condition you have, a specialist in each area. I went on to have a full runner's M.O.T. with Paul and found out some small issues that I was carrying within my body and worked hard to ensure these were all rectified and I feel happier and more confident with my running and have trained more regularly due to a renewed motivation.

Compartment syndrome

What is it?

Exertional compartment syndrome is most common in runners, but not a common injury per se. The muscle mass itself increases in size when running and can reach an increase of 20% compared to its resting state. In some people this increase in size can cause pressure on the vessels that are removing fluid from the muscle, be it blood or lymphatic fluid.

EARLY WARNING SIGNS

- Deep or burning pain in the lateral shin area.
- Weakness and foot drop.

COMMON REASON FOR INJURY

Compartment syndrome that comes on in a chronic sense is one of those that cannot really be avoided, or at least you certainly haven't done anything wrong if you have become injured in this way; it is simply the way your anatomy has developed.

It's worth noting that acute compartment syndrome occurs as a result of an impact, such as in a car crash, for example, rather than a common running injury, but is considered a medical emergency and would require an immediate operation to avoid complications such as nerve damage.

PROGRESSION OF THE INJURY

The inability of the muscle compartment to remove waste fluid or blood results in a build-up of pressure caused by the constant blood supply required for activity. Pain, loss of sensation and sometimes a loss

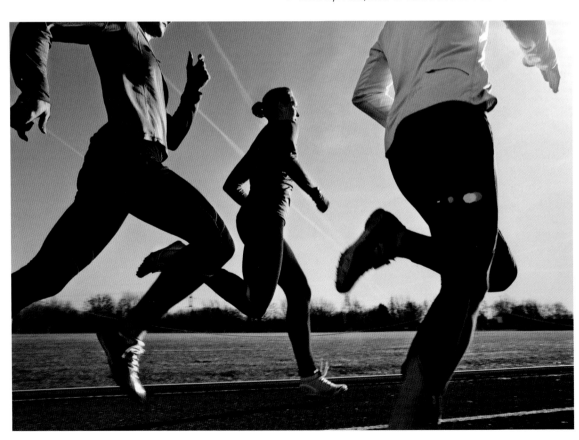

PRACTITIONER PROTOCOL

Assuming you are happy that the patient has exercise-induced compartment syndrome, then proceed with regular and increasingly deep soft tissue massage to the area, including fascial release in all surrounding tissues in an attempt to offload the pressure.

However, do not waste your patient's time; if they need a fasciotomy, then it's best to get them in for the operation and then assist with the rehabilitation afterwards.

In particular, make sure you pay attention to the biomechanics that could be at fault. Look for excessive loading in supination, weakness of tibialis posterior and loss of optimal ankle joints and tarsal joints.

The cause of the issue is often biomechanical and to simply treat without paying attention to these factors is just setting the patient up for a return visit once training is resumed.

of strength can occur (Blackman, 2000). The key here is that, with shin splints or stress fractures, the pain settles very quickly on rest but may be present the next day, but with compartment syndrome, the pain does not settle immediately on rest and can take 10 minutes to an hour before returning to normal. However, there is no pain on the next day.

Pain in the shin area is therefore often confused with shin splints or a stress fracture. This confusion can lead to people using compression garments, which in fact make the problem worse and should be avoided.

SELF-ASSESSMENT

As this injury has potentially hazardous complications if traumatic, I feel it is not sensible to allow someone to self-assess this.

That said, if you have significant pain on the lateral shin when running that seems to get worse and worse and feels like a tight band, you may have exercise-induced compartment syndrome and should seek help. Stop running until you have seen a physiotherapist.

TREATMENT

If you have pain that sits on the lateral aspect of your shin, away from the usual

lower third of the tibia, then consider compartment syndrome and try at first some myofascial release on the area. Myofascial release is a massage technique whereby the fascia (connective tissue) is manipulated away from the muscle structures allowing a freedom of movement between the two. This may help to alleviate the symptoms initially and a period of rest will also help. Strengthening exercises will increase the pain initially so you need both to wait for the pain to settle and consider the surgical options if the issue persists.

In runners, exercise-induced compartment syndrome is treatable with an operation known as a fasciotomy, whereby the fascia (the connective tissue surrounding the muscle) is cut, releasing the muscle, reducing compression and allowing free flow of all substances away from the muscle during exercise.

Manual techniques have worked for this condition and soft tissue massage and fascial release should be attempted first of all. I believe that this injury is often misdiagnosed as shin splints and in many cases the patient is treated for shin splints with soft tissue massage, and the often accidental but positive result is that it works as fascial release. When the 'shin splints' clear up very quickly, this is often the case. Shin splint exercises

I have been running since 2009 and have completed 10 marathons in this time. I have been unfortunate to have suffered from many injuries, from stress fractures, shin splints, sprained ankles, to minor Achilles strains, but, with the help of physiotherapy, have been able to achieve the many marathons I have under my belt.

Last year I suffered from compartment syndrome and had several physio appointments to loosen my calves, this was through soft tissue massages and a form of rolling exercises I was given as homework. With the tight calves and the sheath (that the muscle is in) being smaller than the muscle I was advised to ease back on the running and could continue doing other exercises which

were mainly non-impact, such as aqua jogging, which helped keep up my fitness.

I was prescribed rehab exercises with resistance bands to focus on the glutes, doing lunges, controlled clams and reverse clams. When my shins were totally pain-free I started working on leg strength doing squats and lunges to increase my leg strength. I'm now religious about incorporating strength and conditioning, work and have a programme I follow.

I've learnt the best way to manage an injury is to seek physio help immediately. A niggle might develop into something bigger, which then requires a longer time to heal.

that cause more pain to the area can often be a clue that you are working on the wrong injury and you should report this back to your physio so they can have a rethink.

SELF-TREATMENT
Rest, ice and lateral taping can help. It is important to reduce the inflammation and rest is the best way to do this as the muscle will no longer be filling with blood and lymph fluid, therefore reducing the pressure.

WHAT TO EXPECT FROM A PHYSIOTHERAPIST
The physiotherapist needs to make a judgment call as to whether you have serious acute compartment syndrome, which requires immediate onward referral, or if you have chronic compartment syndrome whereby rest and anti-inflammatory treatments such as ice and ibuprofen are to be used. The likely outcome, however, may be onward referral for a fasciotomy where they cut the tissue that surrounds the muscle to give it more room.

GETTING BACK TO RUNNING
This is difficult to predict because if you manage to get the swelling under control, then as soon as you start to run it may just come straight back again and there are no good predictors for this either way. If the surgical route was required then you will, as with any other surgery, be building the strength back slowly, doing specific exercises to keep soft tissues stretched and at the same time strengthening the foot mechanics to prevent overload of the anterior shin muscles when you do get back to running.

Tibial stress fracture

What is it?

The tibial stress fracture (see page 48 for more detail on stress fractures) is an overuse injury where the stress builds up and goes beyond that of shin splints. The recovery for this is usually at least six weeks of rest, sometimes longer and it is recommended that you avoid any sort of impact. Occasionally, you may

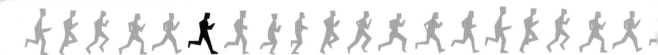

need crutches for the initial period.

It is my experience that runners often come back too early from a stress fracture and can end up with a repeat injury. Six to eight weeks off running is required but you cannot just start running again at the end of the layoff.

The cause of the stress fracture needs to be established first: typically it's caused by overtraining, not taking enough rest or ramping training up too quickly, often in the pursuit of marathon mileage. All too often there is a biomechanical fault, even if the person has been running for several years without issue. The fault can have come about as a build-up of muscle imbalance over time, a fallen arch or chronic tightness in a certain area. This build-up can be multifactorial, in the sense that a new job requiring a new sitting position can be enough to start the process, which becomes magnified once running.

Therefore when you find yourself rehabilitating from a stress fracture, take the time to review old race footage, the images you buy after a race and any coaching videos you might have, and look for areas of weakness, difference from left to right, a dropped shoulder, a tracking knee, a dropped arch etc. You need to take the time to strip back your technique, take on new drills, and strength and conditioning exercises.

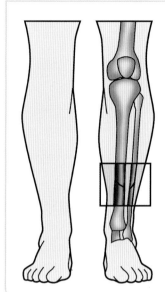

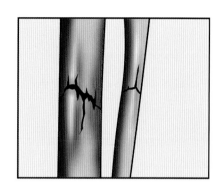

Tibia and fibular stress fracture

EARLY WARNING SIGNS

- Pain on activity, at a specific site within the shin, usually in the lower medial third of the bone
- Pain eases with rest
- Pain does not go away as activity increases, if anything it gets worse.

COMMON REASONS FOR INJURY

People at risk are those with:

- Poor biomechanics
- Weak glutes
- Poor foot posture
- Badly fitting footwear
- Poor running technique
- Those who increase training too quickly
- Overtraining
- Not taking enough rest
- Vitamin D deficiency
- Females that train too hard and do not menstruate
- Post-menopausal women.

The diagnosis is often missed or misdiagnosed by runners who continue on through the pain until it becomes unbearable. There is no shortcut to fixing this problem, regardless of your ability as a runner, you cannot speed up bone healing times.

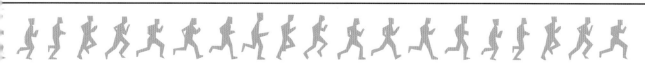

PRACTITIONER PROTOCOL

Use your otherwise redundant ultrasound machine to help with the assessment; turn it up to a high, continuous setting and see if there is pain over the site of injury. If unsure, then send for an MRI scan where possible.

Treatment will depend upon severity, but for completeness opt for non-weight bearing until you have a firm diagnosis.

- Speed recovery with crutches or an orthopedic support or both
- Use the assessment session to look at general strength and conditioning of the runner, check for core strength, glute activation, hamstring equality and hip flexor tightness
- Set a programme around your findings with home exercises that do not load the injured foot
- Set aqua jogging sessions and a full series of strength and conditioning exercises specific to running to ensure that the runner can return to full fitness as quickly as possible post recovery.

PROGRESSION OF THE INJURY

This is often misdiagnosed as shin splints and this delays the process of rest that is required. Nothing will improve a tibial stress fracture quicker than rest over six weeks, but taking a calcium supplement may help strengthen the bone tissue and ensure that your nutrition is optimized.

SELF-ASSESSMENT

Run your hand down your shin, until you feel the area that is clearly in the most pain. Press quite firmly about three inches away from the area of pain, onto the shin bone. Gradually press along the bone getting closer and closer to the site of pain. If you feel little or no pain until you are directly over the injury site, or only slight passed it, but immense pain directly over the injury, this is typical of a stress fracture.

More diffuse pain and swelling, whilst not a clear sign that this is a lesser injury, is less likely to be a stress fracture than pinpoint, very specific acute pain.

TREATMENT

Treatment is usually via rest and, in the worst cases, using crutches to ensure that no loading goes through the bone at all for six weeks.

You will be well advised to spend the time resting your leg, engaging in Pilates and other core strength activities to ensure you have good transverse abdominal recruitment and a strong core. Work on your hip abductors and adductors and hamstring/glute recruitment.

SELF-TREATMENT

As with other bone injuries mentioned earlier, the exercises you are able to do are focused on ameliorating the potential weakness that led to this injury and ensuring that you come back to running a stronger all-round athlete. Therefore, choose these exercises: Towel grabbing (strength), page 167, Calf (stretch), page 168, Soleus (stretch), page 168, The clam – hip abduction/rotation (strength), page 173, Hamstrings (strength), page 174, Glute activation (strength), page 175 and Core muscles (strength), page 176.

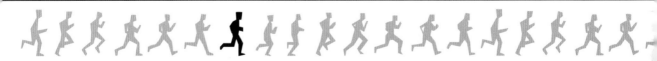

WHAT TO EXPECT FROM A PHYSIOTHERAPIST

For assessment purposes, your physio will ask a number of relevant questions which will give them the cues needed to make their diagnosis. To confirm their diagnosis, they will likely use therapeutic ultrasound, which will produce sound waves that unsettle the stress fracture and cause pain. Using the device on healthy bone or other soft tissue won't cause pain.

After putting ultrasound gel on both shins, your physio will slowly move the device back and forth over each shin. You should feel no pain on the good shin. On the sore shin, however, if you feeling pain over the site of the injury this points to a stem fracture. X-rays aren't particularly useful until after at least four weeks from the original injury so MRI scans are used to confirm the diagnosis. Typically, a physio would advise you to wear an orthopaedic boot for six weeks and in extremely bad cases, crutches must be used as well.

GETTING BACK TO RUNNING

After a stress fracture, the focus should be on cross training initially, with 80–90% of your time doing non-running activities. During this phase you can aqua jog as much as you like and, if you can, use anti-gravity treadmills that will allow you to spend some time on a treadmill, but with as little as a few per cent of your body weight being transferred through your injured limb.

Aqua jogging for the six weeks is recommended, before starting back on the cross trainer and eventually diluting your percentages on the cross trainer in favour of increasing bouts of running on soft ground. Your final transition will be back to the track or pavement.

CLIENT STORY: PHIL, 32

I first noticed a pain in my shin when running on hard surfaces. It felt like a sharp stabbing pain at first, then a full ache after the run. I continued to run with the pain, assuming it was just referral pain from tight calves but I had to stop when the pain became intense and worse after running, even when the leg wasn't weight bearing. Night pain was also prominent in the days before diagnosis with a dull ache felt in the shin area periodically during sleep.

I then saw Paul who diagnosed a stress fracture after key examinations of the leg and the symptoms that I described. Initial rehabilitation was to avoid any weight bearing activity on the injured leg. The length of time estimated for recovery was six weeks and this involved a programme of rehabilitation exercises that were designed to reduce the inflammation around the injury and ultimately address the imbalances that caused it to occur in the first instance. A series of

tests by Paul revealed weaknesses in both the glute and hamstring and poor biomechanics through the foot strike in the injured leg.

Regular breaking down of the scar tissue around the injury site was important towards the end of rehabilitation to ensure a successful transition back to training when ready.

Non weight-bearing exercise was crucial to maintain aerobic fitness during the injury period and this was carried out in the form of aqua jogging or pool running.

Upon return to running again, a gradual introduction to weight-bearing exercise was implemented on soft flat surfaces. The key to ensuring the injury doesn't return is to continue to address the weaknesses diagnosed in both biomechanics and key muscle groups. The exercises prescribed during rehabilitation needed to be carried out regularly and when returning to normal training to limit re-injury.

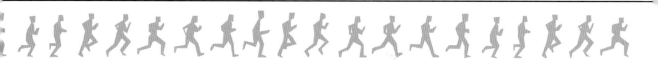

CHAPTER 4

THE KNEE

A huge percentage of runners complain of knee pain and this is the most common injury I will treat all year round. There is definitely a spike in visitors with knee pain between February and May when runners are training for the spring marathons. It would seem that anecdotally the knee of a new runner will start to cause pain once the mileage creeps over 15–20 miles per week, whereas the first-time marathon runner, with a background in running, will present with knee pain after the 14–16 mile run stage of the programme.

My suspicion is that almost all runners will experience knee pain at some point in their lives, but for many, a foam roller, a little rest and some new trainers will resolve or manage the issue. However, for those with some biomechanical issues, the knee will cause them a great deal of angst and will require a review of everything from hip strength to footwear choice.

I am not in agreement with the contention that running creates knee pain. Many people walk around in inappropriate, unsupportive footwear, with a weak set of core muscles and poor knee alignment, which is only discovered when they decide to run. The problem here is someone needs to run in order to find their knee pain earlier than old age will.

The knee is a wonderfully complex and injury-prone joint, with its controlling muscles largely based at the hip and its foundations and stability coming from the highly mobile foot and ankle joint. The poor knee is caught between the weak glutes and the wobbly ankles, with little resistance or defence against unwanted movement. The knee demands good strength at the hip and core and incredible balance and alignment at the ankle. With these two parameters in place the hip, knee and ankle joints can sit on top of one another in a nice functional line, largely impervious to injury.

The following is a list of common running knee injuries. There are so many subtle diagnoses of knee injury, but this list is limited to the most common injuries I see in clinic.

- ITB friction syndrome
- Patellofemoral pain syndrome (PFPS, also known as runner's knee)
- Patella tendinopathy
- Chondromalacia patellae
- Meniscus cartilage injury
- Pes anserinus bursitis
- Osgood-Schlatter disease
- Fat pad impingement/Hoffa's fat pad
- Medial collateral ligament (MCL) and Lateral collateral ligament (LCL)
- Anterior cruciate ligament (ACL) and Posterior collateral ligament (PCL).

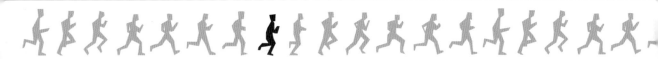

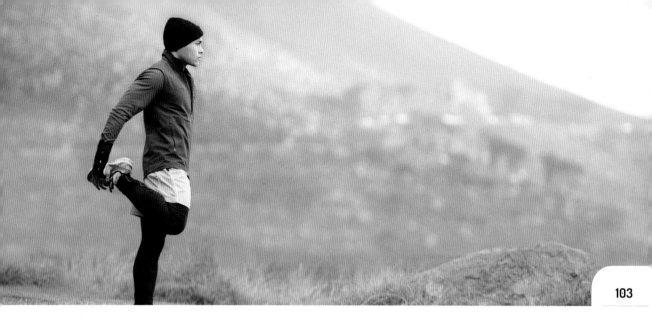

ITB friction syndrome

What is it?

Iliotibial band (ITB) friction syndrome is one of the most common chronic running injuries. I suspect that a great many of you will have already experienced it. It can be confused or co-exist with patellofemoral pain syndrome (PFPS) (see page 110) and so the information contained in this section refers to both conditions. The subtle differences are outlined in the short section on PFPS.

The ITB is the band that travels from the lateral hip down to the knee, controlled by two muscles, the Tensor fascia latae (TFL) and gluteus maximus (glute max) helping to keep the knee aligned and to control unwanted movement.

The pain comes about because the ITB is being overworked in an attempt to keep the knee alignment true and the two controlling muscles tighten. The ITB therefore gets pulled tight against the lateral knee joint and this is where the friction can occur.

I read and hear advice about foam rolling the ITB all the time, and many do this prophylactically as a defence mechanism. The issue is that the ITB is made of very tough, robust, inflexible material, which is no more likely to lengthen through foam rolling, than the desk I sit at to write this book. It's a myth that the ITB can be stretched or lengthened in any way.

However, there is hope, as the muscles TFL and glute max can be stretched, if only a little, but this can create sufficient 'slack' to be beneficial. The root cause as to why the ITB is being stressed through tension should be the focus of the treatment and management for this injury.

EARLY WARNING SIGNS

- Pain over the lateral aspect of the knee when running
- This pain will stop when you stop running
- Pain going downstairs but little or no pain going upstairs
- Pain will worsen with movement, especially running and continue to get worse until you stop running.

COMMON REASONS FOR INJURY

- A narrow stride width
- Increasing your running mileage too quickly
- Poor footwear choice; take the time to have a running shoe properly fitted following an assessment in a running shop
- Loss of core strength
- Poor hip control/strength.

THE KNEE

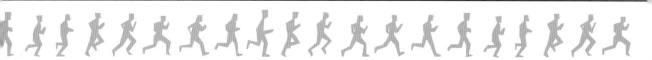

PROGRESSION OF THE INJURY

The pain becomes unremitting, having started out as a pain only felt when running. The pain is felt as a constant ache behind the kneecap as the lateral pull of the ITB has started to cause a closely related injury called Patellofemoral pain syndrome. You will feel pain on walking and there can also be a throbbing at rest due to inflammation. At this point, there is very little chance of you running.

SELF-ASSESSMENT

Feel the lateral aspect of your knee, if there is pain and tenderness over this outside area, which seems to be worse with movement, especially going downstairs, then you are halfway to your diagnosis.

Stand in front of a full-length mirror and perform a single leg squat on the non-affected side, to see if your knee travels inwards over the midline. Now assess the painful side and see if there is more or less travel. A tight ITB may mean that this tests produces a 'false negative', meaning you pass the text due to overtightening of these structures.

Now perform the Tensor fascia latae (stretch) (p. 178), three times for 45 seconds. Repeat the test. This time, if there is less pain and the knee travels farther, you have gone a long way to diagnosing yourself with ITB syndrome, but this will need confirming in clinic by a trained physiotherapist.

TREATMENT

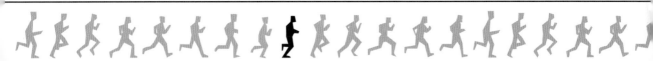

One of the treatment options is to release TFL, this can be done almost instantly with some trigger point work (pushing in with your thumbs to slow the blood supply, therefore starving the muscle of the oxygen and calcium it needs to contract). With a stretch straight after the trigger point work, you can give a release to the TFL and therefore the ITB. This is where treatment and assessment can overlap, as a physio may like to watch the person once again on the single leg squat and maybe even the treadmill to see the difference in control whilst there is less tension in the ITB.

This way, even if you've been partially treated, the physio can take away the natural scaffolding (tight TFL) and then see the true mechanics of the running gait and get a much clearer picture of your injury.

After this assessment on the treadmill, I then reassess the ITB tension to see if some, or all, has returned. This gives me an idea as to how rapidly the treatments I provide are losing their effects and I can cross reference this with their clinical picture. For example, if the pain was coming on during the first five minutes of a run, I can begin to see this for myself as part of my test-retest protocol.

If, during this assessment, it becomes clear that you are working very hard to stabilize the knee via the foot and ankle, the work trigger pointing TFL is unlikely to change the picture. In this instance it is time to consider footwear, strength and potentially an insert into the shoe, perhaps only for an initial period to support the failing mechanics of the foot and ankle.

There is so much to look at: the rotation of your femur, the strength of the smaller glutes (minimus and medius) and then there is your core strength, (which if compromised will prevent good mechanics when running despite you having the strongest of glutes), good foot and ankle balance and a relatively relaxed ITB.

At the risk of blinding you with all these variables, it would seem that this (the most common of runners' complaints), could be so totally different from person to person, with seemingly the same symptoms. It is therefore not reasonable to simply keep punishing yourself with a foam roller, day in day out and hope for the best. Diagnosis takes time, the recovery can be very quick with the right diagnosis, so this is an injury worth the time and money to see an experienced professional.

What we are aiming for at the knee is good alignment and with that a correctly tracking patella (kneecap). This is the ability of the structures that surround the knee to keep the kneecap on course as it slides up and down the deep groove in the thigh bone during knee flexion and extension.

Strength and conditioning training is the key to this, which must be functional. The training to support a knee can be static initially, such as the clam. Within a matter of weeks you will notice that you can hold your knee plumb straight and get your knee bend below 90 degrees, way past what you need for running. As your strength improves, so does your knee control.

SELF-TREATMENT

Perform the following exercises: Single leg balance, p. 171, The clam – hip abduction/rotation (strength), p. 173, Hip adductors (stretch), p. 174, Glute activation (strength), p. 175, Core muscles (strength), p. 176, Glutes (stretch), p. 177, ITB Tensor fascia latae (stretch) p. 178 and Side step with squat (strength), p. 179.

A trick that I like to use for patella tracking is to tape the knee during the early stages of rehabilitation. Kinesiology tape is my preferred product as I can produce tension where I need it to be tight around the joint and allow the natural stretch of the tape to remain where it's not. This means you can anchor the tape below the kneecap and stretch it tight as it passes the curve of the patella, adhere it there and then relax the tape once more to anchor to the thigh.

The result of the first piece of tape should look like the top photo, close to the patella and on a slightly bent knee. The second piece of tape is applied so it splits the knee cap and pulls tight around the patella. The third peice is applied the other way around so it encases the patella. The final peice of tape is cut specifically to go around the base of the patella to give final support and also prevent any loose ends coming free.

If the taping is applied and you run pretty much pain free, then this will show you the end result of your physiotherapy and rehabilitation exercises. The focus should now be on getting the biomechanics and strength to take over the work of the tape and return to a pain-free/tape-free existence.

WHAT TO EXPECT FROM A PHYSIOTHERAPIST

I like to look at my patient running on the treadmill initially. Whilst this isn't the exact replica of the running action whilst out on the road or track, it's a close second when it comes to analysis. By

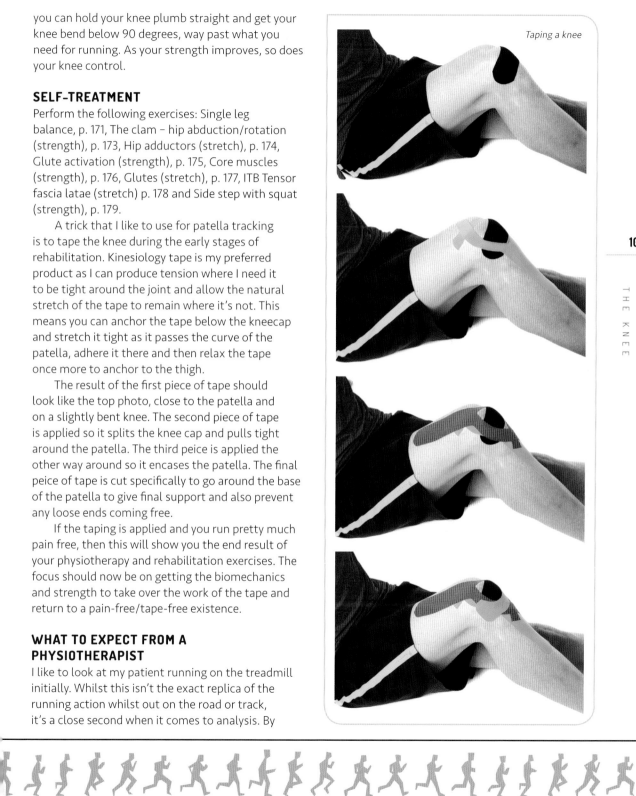

Taping a knee

looking in turn at the foot and ankle through each stride, I move then to focus on the knee position as it travels through a gait cycle and lastly, the hip position. From this information a physio can identify significant differences from left to right and also rate this against what is considered 'normal'.

The physiotherapist will have learned the key areas to assess. He or she will initially look at the hip and leg position in mid-stance (a video freeze frame during gait analysis). Looking from the front, they want to assess for FADDIR, which is a hip that is flexed, adducted and internally rotated. This demonstrates weakness in the abductors and external hip rotators, with tightness in the hip flexors and adductors. The femur has no option but to roll inwards causing patella mis-tracking.

Physios use the single leg squat a lot in diagnoses of knee pain. With approximately 3–5 reps, the physio will assess how the person is working to try to maintain knee alignment and their success or failure in doing so.

The test is a functional one, looking at movement patterns. This is a great diagnostic tool for the physio looking at a patient for the first time, but let them know if you've visited another physio before. The assessment becomes less meaningful if the individual has sought advice from a number of therapists and has been working on the strength of their single leg squat for five weeks. This will mean that you may have become good at the art of performing a single leg squat with good form, which takes away an analysis tool as part of the

assessment procedure and its relevance to diagnosis. What a physio is looking for is deviation from the central line. The knee falling inwards as the leg bends, the foot and ankle over-pronating, the pelvic alignment being lost. All this information helps the physiotherapist to make informed judgments about where the weakness might lie.

Once your physio has assessed the single leg squat and possibly taken some video on the treadmill, he or she will start to build a picture of where the weakness might be. They will then perform a thorough assessment on the treatment couch and assess each part of the functional chain in turn.

There are two muscles called the gluteus medius and gluteus minimus that perform a key role in these biomechanics and can be germane to a whole host of injuries, so they need some explanation.

These muscles are key abductors and medial rotators of the hip (when the hip is flexed); they act as stabilizers during the gait cycle to prevent the opposite hip from dropping as it swings through, and abduct as the controlling leg swings through to ensure you don't knock your knees together.

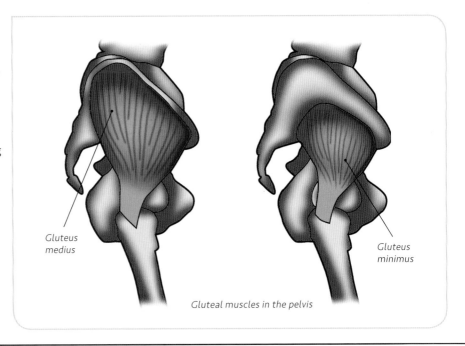

Gluteus medius

Gluteus minimus

Gluteal muscles in the pelvis

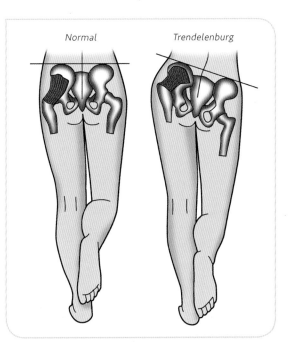

Normal   Trendelenburg

These two muscles are of utmost importance in knee control and keeping the pelvic alignment during the gait cycle. Without strength in the abductors, you end up with a pelvis that is known as 'Trendelenburg' (see figure below) where the pelvis and therefore the hip/leg drops during the swing phase of the gait cycle.

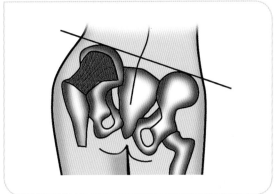

PRACTITIONER PROTOCOL

As the ITB has no contractile portion and has the tensile strength of steel, you will not manipulate this with any treatment. The contractile portions of tensor fascia lata and gluteus maximus can, however, be treated successfully, and trigger point release to TFL especially will significantly increase the range of motion (ROM) of the lateral quadrant.

However, with the loss of tension comes a functional error in knee control, so strength training for the glute minimus, medius and maximus is imperative as well as hip hitching and more advanced TFL strengthening including a leg swing to make it more running specific. Ankle proprioception and core strength make for a very well rounded protocol, which if successful, should resolve ITBS in a matter of weeks.

SSTM to the quads, working into the specific muscle groups that showed up as tight on assessment. I do not subscribe to the notion that VMO can be individually trained but that doesn't mean that inner range quads exercises are not part of the protocol (Inner range quad, page 181). Single leg squats performed with increasing depth over the weeks of rehabilitation, starting with minimal movement over a few centimetres' depth at first, working slowly up to a 65-degree bend within a few weeks. Gain early control first then develop the range of motion alongside the attained abduction and glute max strength.

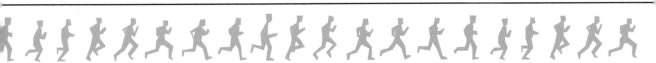

In response your knees may drift towards the midline and cause many of the issues discussed in this chapter, and you will experience pain both laterally on the knee, laterally at the hip and in the lower back.

The clam is one of the exercises of choice as it works both the glute medius and minimus but also the hip rotators, however, it does not provide the functional element of strength which the single leg squat, quarter turn squat jumps (single leg) or similar types of drill do.

GETTING BACK TO RUNNING

If you are able to run pain-free with the tape, it's a good idea to continue to run, maintain the strength in the areas that have built up over months of training and do the additional work to strengthen your weaker muscle groups. You will then be able to remove the tape and rely on your own physiology once more.

There is one other factor we need to consider, the hip flexion/extension balance. If the hip is experiencing resistance into extension, then the hip will remain in some degree of flexion throughout the gait cycle, this in turn means the knee has to remain slightly flexed at all times. If the knee remains flexed then there is a constant and unremitting pull on the patella into the femur and the result is wear and tear. Add to this patella tracking issues and there is simply no respite from the injury cause. You need to make sure that you have adequate hip extension, the normal value for which is 10–15 degrees. Check this by laying face down on the ground and lift up your leg, if you can raise it high enough to put a pillow under your thigh, then you have 'normal' muscle range.

CLIENT STORY: JILL, 49

I am a full-time doctor, and mother of four children aged between 12 and 16. I started running when my youngest child was three and I needed to get fit again. Having always done a lot of sport I needed to exercise when the kids and husband were asleep so as to impact as little as possible on family life – and running was the cheapest and most accessible choice. I immediately fell in love with it. I ran a few half marathons without proper training, including a PB of 1hr 41mins, but it wasn't until moving to Australia four years ago that running became a big part of social and family life. The whole family now runs, and my main social life out of work is with my running mates, who have proven to be the most supportive, encouraging, loyal and fantastic friends.

My injury occurred shortly after running my first marathon in Melbourne in October 2013 (3hr 49min). I loved every minute – from the early morning pre-work training runs, right up to the last km of the marathon (actually my fastest km!). I could not wait to run another one. Having religiously read the marathon training schedules, unfortunately, I forgot to read the post-race instructions. Buoyed up by adrenaline, after a day of rest I continued as if nothing had changed – still running 15 to 20k a day.

Two weeks later, in the middle of a normal run, completely out of the blue, a terrible pain started in my knee – it seemed to get worse every time I lifted my leg, and after less than 1k I could hardly walk. I really felt as though something bad had happened. I hobbled home and spent the next few weeks icing, resting, trying to run, trying to walk, and the pain just got worse. I dusted off my bike, and so began six months of cycling frantically to maintain some level of fitness. As I am a radiologist I quickly got myself an ultrasound and MRI – both showing classic ITB syndrome.

The next few months were spent in and out of depression – I had Googled ITB syndrome and set myself on a self-prescribed course of rolling, strength exercises, rest, icing, trying to run, cycling

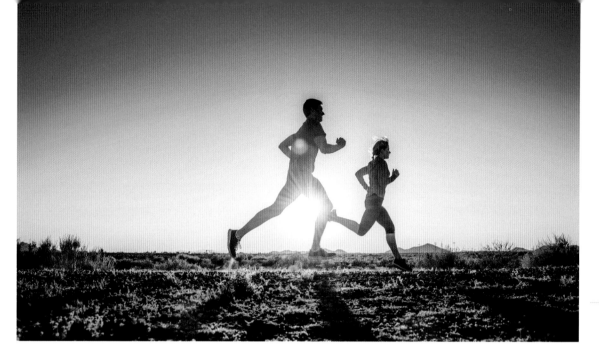

etc. At its intermittent worst I could hardly walk the 1.5k into town from home. I was very down and thought I may never run again. I even saw an orthopaedic surgeon, who threatened various surgical procedures and also was fairly pessimistic about me ever running another marathon. If it wasn't for my fabulous group of friends who never gave up on me, and who even dusted off their own bikes to join me out riding, I am not sure that I would have managed to stay positive.

A planned flying visit back to London to visit family, and further desperation led me to Physio&Therapy UK, an email address and link I had seen in Runner's World. I emailed and set up an appointment to be assessed.

The appointment in April 2014 was the turning point in my recovery. A detailed examination from pretty much top to bottom, took 90 minutes, from fitness to flexibility, strength to weakness – and that assessment highlighted a number of weaknesses – despite four months of having fairly religiously followed daily exercises I had never done before, trying to strengthen hips, core, even up dominant and non-dominant sides, etc. It turned out that without knowing I had a huge amount more work to do. I was directed round the corner to get kitted out with properly fitting running shoes, was given a targeted personalized rehabilitation regime to get going on. Back on the plane that evening I could not wait to start. My physio emailed details including diagrams of my regimen so there were no excuses about forgetting.

The results were quite astonishing and within a month I had struggled back up to running a slow 5k. After that, improvement was rapid and return to fitness was thereafter much, much quicker than I had imagined. No one was more surprised than myself when in October 2014, I lined up again for the start of the Melbourne marathon. I managed to knock 8 minutes off my PB to finish in 3hr 41min.

My strength, core exercise routine is now a daily part of my training. I feel like I am a stronger, better, healthier runner. So far, ITB syndrome has not reared its ugly head again, and I am training now to run the Boston Marathon in April, having been lucky enough to qualify. I am hoping that my new holistic approach to running will keep me injury-free.

Patellofemoral pain syndrome (PFPS or Runner's Knee)

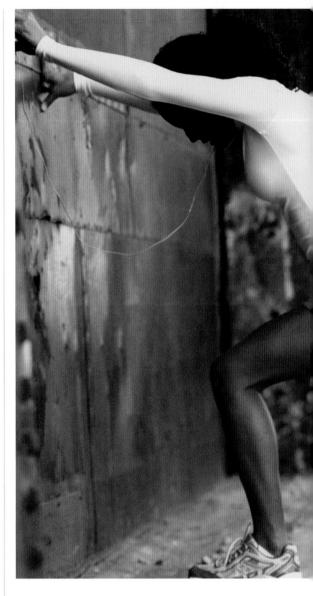

A caveat here. The overlap of information in this section and the previous one on the ITB is huge. I have limited this to a small section as a result, in the hope that you will see them as interchangeable diagnosis and treatment strategies. If you see a physiotherapist, it is likely he or she will be treating both as a rule anyway. The following few words are merely to help you to understand the differences and I urge you to read both sections.

What is it?

PFPS is as common if not slightly more so than ITB friction syndrome. The fact is that one often exists with the other anyway and the diagnostic process for ITB can be almost exactly the same. In fact, the similarities of cause are astonishingly close. There is more in terms of wear and tear for PFPS as it's the approximation of two joint surfaces, causing friction and damage over time if left.

The telltale sign a physio will be looking for when assessing a patient is when they mention pain laterally or anteriorly behind the patella. The anterior knee pain is due to pain between the inner surface of the patella (kneecap) and the base of your thigh bone. PFPS stands for the patellafemoral (thigh bone) pain syndrome: so basically, knee cap overload within its groove on the femur. This happens because of poor patella tracking within the femoral groove. When you have poor tracking the ITB pulls tightly against the bone as it passes over the lateral knee joint and causes friction at that site.

There is a simple diagnostic test we can do as physiotherapists, whereby we release the tensor fascia latae muscle (TFL – a hip flexor sitting just underneath your jeans coin pocket) by applying pressure and then a stretch to this muscle, as it is the key contractile portion of the ITB. By releasing the TFL, it is easy to re-test the patient for range of movement and also pain reduction when walking or performing functional testing. A more effective assessment is for the patient to go on a treadmill after the kinesiology tape has been used to fix the patella in place and see if this makes for a less painful run. With the adjustment of poor tracking of the patella, the patient can feel immediate relief.

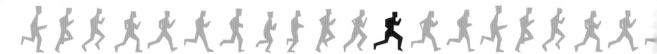

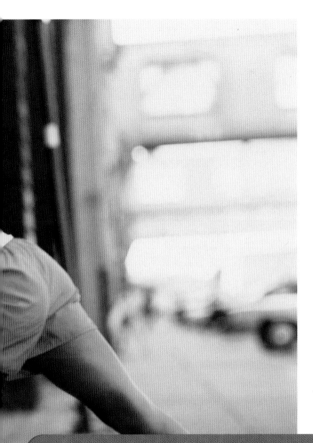

It is not uncommon for runners with PFPS to spend weeks in tape so they can continue to run whilst building up the muscle strength in order to offer a more natural support to the knee. Physiotherapy time is taken addressing the core issues, lengthening structures where possible and not only prescribing the rehab schedule but the training plan as well.

It is rare that a runner presents with either PFPS or ITB friction syndrome and is unable to complete his or her chosen race or goal.

SELF-ASSESSMENT

Pain in the anterior knee, with pain felt in behind the kneecap. With your legs out straight and the patella relaxed, try placing a small but increasing amount of pressure down over the kneecap, this will be more painful on the injured side.

You can also try contracting your quads muscles (front of thigh) with the legs straight and relaxed as above, looking out for an increased pain on the injured side.

Lastly, try performing a single leg squat, five or six times without stopping to balance yourself, and see if the pain increases on the injured side.

PRACTITIONER PROTOCOL

Similar to the treatment for ITBS, the benefits to the patient are to prevent the mis-tracking of the patella through strength training for the glute minimus, medius and maximus. Be sure to include hip hitching and more advanced TFL strengthening including a leg swing to make it more running specific. Ankle proprioception and core strength make for a very well rounded protocol.

SSTM to the quads, working into the specific muscle groups that showed up as tight on assessment. I do not subscribe to the notion that VMO can be individually trained but that doesn't mean that inner range quads exercises are not part of the protocol (see Inner range quad, page 181). Single leg squats performed with increasing depth over the weeks of rehabilitation, starting with minimal movement over a few centimetres' depth at first, working slowly up to a 65-degree bend within a few weeks. Gain early control first, then develop the range of motion alongside the attained abduction and glute max strength.

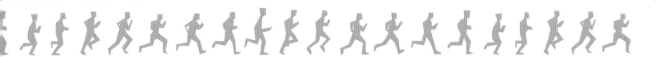

Patella tendinopathy

What is it?

This is the tendon that runs from the kneecap through to the tibial tuberosity on the lower leg bone (the tibia) and serves as the tendinous attachment for the quadriceps muscle. The patella is actually a floating bone within the tendon material and, in theory, as this 'tendon' runs from bone to bone it should correctly be called a ligament, but most still refer to it as the patellar tendon.

When the tendon becomes inflamed, much like an Achilles tendinopathy, you get a very similar kind of damage to the collagen, causing pain and loss of optimal performance, not only for the patella itself but its joint with the femur (patellofemoral joint) and the knee joint itself. Pain will cause the body to look for less uncomfortable ways to move and this can create issues elsewhere as you try to continue to run through it.

This injury is also known as Jumper's Knee and is associated with sports that have a lot of bounding and explosive movements with the legs. Track running potentially puts a runner at more risk than less explosive road running.

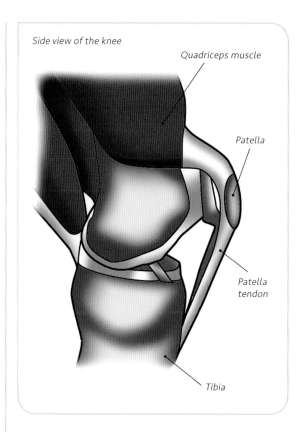

Side view of the knee

Quadriceps muscle

Patella

Patella tendon

Tibia

EARLY WARNING SIGNS

- Pain just below the kneecap, specifically when the quadriceps muscle is being used, e.g. walking upstairs
- Stiffness in the anterior knee first thing
- Tight quadriceps muscles
- Unable to kneel.

COMMON REASONS FOR INJURY

For the majority of runners, this will be after doing some additional training around their usual running programme, such as hill sprints, strength and conditioning training in the gym, or plyometric training and drills.

It can also happen when trainers are coming to the end of their lifespan, a sudden increase in training load and also from micro trauma as a result of doing something else, e.g. running again after a skiing holiday.

PROGRESSION OF THE INJURY

The usual course of things starts with the onset of pain, stiffness, and loss of strength in that limb. As you continue to use the tendon these symptoms will get worse. The soreness could be worse during the night or first thing in the morning, and the tendon can get tender, red, and inflamed.

There are four key progressive categories of patella tendon injury, starting at the lowest level as a reactive tendinopathy, which if left untreated will turn into tendon disrepair. Most often you will fit into the first two categories and prognosis is excellent with the right treatment. However, if you continue to run and ignore the signs and symptoms, you could end up with a degenerative tendon or worse still, a ruptured tendon.

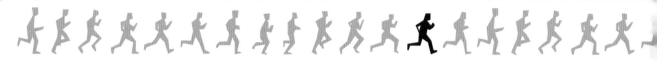

SELF-ASSESSMENT

Pain felt specifically at the tendon that travels from the lowest part of the knee cap to the shinbone immediately below it, and tenderness on touching this area, at the base of your kneecap, plus pain in this specific area when performing a squat, will suggest this as a diagnosis.

Stand with your feet a shoulder-width apart and squat down. Pain on the affected side in the specific area just below the knee is a positive test. Try performing a Single leg squat (strength), page 175, to see if the pain intensifies.

TREATMENT

Treatment is to initially rest from the aggravating activity, and then start with appropriate loading of the tendon. Reduce tension in the quadriceps muscle through soft tissue massage and where appropriate using a technique referred to throughout this book, deep transverse frictions (DTF). DTF is a sawing-like action of the fingertips or thumb over the injured tendon to stimulate the cell growth within the structure and accelerate the healing process.

SELF-TREATMENT

Appropriate loading of the tendon is of particular importance, as with other tendons in this book, starting with isometric loading, then HSR, and moving onto eccentric loading as shown. For this you will need to use a 30–45 degree board (sold online as calf stretchers) allowing you to do a decline squat as pictured, right. These should be performed as follows:

- Stand on a decline board, balancing on the injured leg
- Slowly lower yourself down taking 6–10 seconds
- Place your non-injured leg on the board and use this leg to push you back to the start position
- Repeat 15 times x 3 on alternate days
- After 4 weeks increase the resistance using a back pack with some weight inside, and perform 10 reps x 4
- After 4 weeks of 10 reps, increase the weight and repeat 6 times x 4.

In addition, choose the following exercises: The clam – hip abduction/rotation (strength), page 173, Hip flexors (stretch), page 173, Single leg squat (strength), page 175, Glute activation (strength) page 175 and Quads stretch, page 182.

WHAT TO EXPECT FROM A PHYSIOTHERAPIST

When you see a physiotherapist, you should expect to undergo a full examination of the knee, foot mechanics and pelvic stability; and tests for muscle length, strength and also joint movement and alignment.

Once this information has been processed then the cause of the stress to the patella tendon can be surmised as either a biomechanical issue or overuse injury. The treatments of soft tissue work and exercise prescription will not vary greatly, but the cause of the injury must be addressed for you to have a full recovery, so expect plenty of functional testing on your visit.

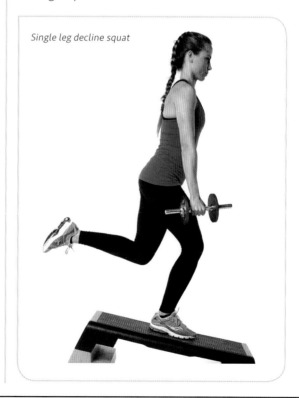

Single leg decline squat

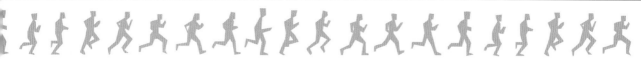

PRACTITIONER PROTOCOL

It's important to take the tension out of the quads, just like with the patella fat pad impingement.

- SSTM to rectus femoris but also to the vastus lateralis and vastus medialis aims to reduce the pull on the patella tendon. Stretches can be performed as well, so long as irritation does not increase as a result, and massage can be a great early management of the tension
- DTF to the patella tendon
- Taping to offload the patella
- Inner range quads, abduction strength (Hip adductors (stretch), page 174, Inner range quad, page 181, and Quads stretch, page 182)
- Shockwave therapy to the tendon 500 shocks at 1.5htz, 10 per second, followed by 2000 shocks at 2.5htz at 10 per second, 3–4 sessions at 7-day intervals.

CLIENT STORY: ROSSCO, 25

I am an elite level runner having competed at Olympic level over 1500m. Having suffered with injury through my career like so many, I have always worked hard to find a speedy resolution to the issue and to do this I have surrounded myself with some top professionals in the industry. One such professional is Paul Hobrough who I have been fortunate to be able to see where I train in London and also back home in the North East as he has clinics in both locations.

I had been working hard at a training camp in Kenya and therefore running on some different road and track surfaces as a result, not to mention altitude, so you can understand that I found it easy to justify a slight niggle in one of my knees and assume it would return to normal on my return home. How wrong I was. The pain was dull and

barely noticeable at first, plus only when I ran. After a week it was pretty much there all the time and much worse if I tried to run.

I went to see Paul and with a few simple tests he explained that my patella tendon was the issue, and set about using treatments that included soft tissue manipulation, kneecap taping and eventually some shockwave therapy. I noticed the improvement immediately the treatment started, getting better every day and once the shockwave therapy started I was having significant periods of time totally pain free.

The treatments worked and I haven't had any reoccurrence of the issue. I have continued to develop my strength and conditioning training to strengthen the whole leg and pelvis to ensure my pending trip to Kenya does not create the same issue.

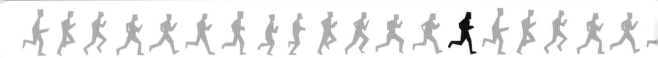

In addition to this, a well-equipped physiotherapy clinic will offer you shockwave therapy (see page 37). With success rates ranging from 65–91% it's clear why shockwave therapy is fast becoming the leading treatment for musculoskeletal disorders, with more and more injuries being added to the approved list as new research is presented.

GETTING BACK TO RUNNING

The road back to running will vary depending upon the amount of time you have had the injury and the treatment options available to you. Shockwave therapy will speed the process and when combined with the eccentric loading, you could find yourself sufficiently pain-free in a matter of weeks.

Start off with rehabilitation runs of 3 minutes in duration x 5, stopping to stretch the quad (Quads stretch, page 182) during the breaks. Rest for 2 days then try 5 x 4 minutes, rest for 2 days then increase the runs to 5 minutes. Continue with this until 7-minute runs are possible then start to reduce the set numbers as the time increases until you are running 3 x 10 minutes, then 2 x 15 min and 2 x 20 minutes. From here you can start to access your usual training programme again.

Chondromalacia patellae

What is it?

Chondromalacia patellae is an injury found in young athletes. It is more common in girls and is different to PFPS because there is no cartilage damage. The cause is similar to that of PFPS, often a weakness in the muscles at the lateral hip, which means the knee drops in medially at mid-stance. The result is inflammation caused by a tight ITB and overuse, misalignment, core instability weakness, and most commonly patellar mis-tracking.

EARLY WARNING SIGNS

- Painful knees during and after exercise
- The pain is felt behind the kneecap, under the kneecap and sometimes to the side of the knee
- Rest eases the pain, but inflammation can cause a constant ache.

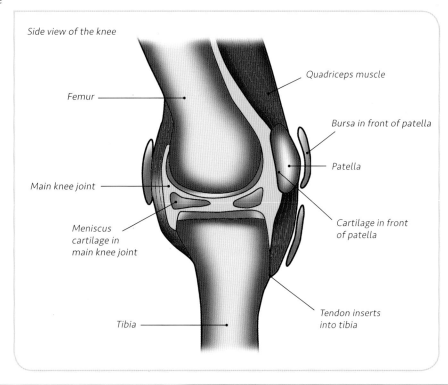

Side view of the knee

Quadriceps muscle

Femur

Bursa in front of patella

Patella

Main knee joint

Meniscus cartilage in main knee joint

Cartilage in front of patella

Tibia

Tendon inserts into tibia

COMMON REASONS FOR INJURY

Adolescents grow in bursts and this changes the biomechanics of their lower limbs, muscles need to adjust to the additional length and strength requirements.

There is a higher incidence of young females suffering with chondromalacia patella because females generally have a higher degree of valgus knee, whereby the knee comes in across the midline on walking, running and squatting. This stress causes tension in the ITB and mis-tracking of the patella; the result is pain.

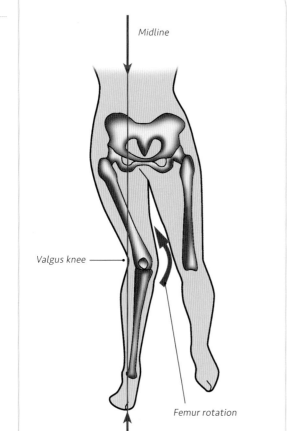

Midline

Valgus knee

Femur rotation

PROGRESSION OF THE INJURY

The progression is largely related to usage; like PFPS, the more you use the knee and load it during running, the worse it will get. Rest will restore the symptoms to a more manageable level.

SELF-ASSESSMENT

Pain in the anterior knee, with pain felt behind the kneecap (patella) are the indicators. With your legs out straight and the patella relaxed, try placing a small but increasing amount of pressure down over the kneecap, this will be more painful on the injured side. You can also try contracting your quads muscles (front of thigh) with the legs straight and relaxed as above, looking for an increased pain on the injured side.

Stand in front of a full-length mirror and perform a single leg squat on the non-affected side, to see if your knee travels inwards over the midline.

Lastly, try performing a single leg squat five or six times without stopping to balance yourself, and see if the pain increases on the injured side.

TREATMENT

The treatment is broadly the same as for PFPS: offload the joint surfaces through reducing the pull of the kneecap laterally through tight structures such as ITB, aid the alignment of the knee with the same exercises as per PFPS and work on functional strength with such exercises as the single leg squat, ensuring that you start with very small movements and graduate slowly into deep squats.

SELF-TREATMENT

Follow exercises: Single leg balance, page 171, The clam – hip abduction/rotation (strength), page 173, Hip adductors (stretch), page 174, Single leg squat (strength), page 175, Glute activation (strength), page 175 and ITB Tensor fascia latae (stretch), page 178.

WHAT TO EXPECT FROM A PHYSIOTHERAPIST

When you see a physiotherapist for chondromalacia patella, you may be seeing one for the first time as

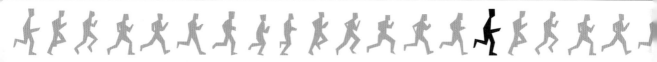

PRACTITIONER PROTOCOL

Similar to the treatment for ITBS and PFPS, however, in most cases you will be faced with a younger patient and therefore giving too many exercises will be pointless. (Often it is for the older client as well, but with a good older runner, the compliance is usually better.)

The aim is to prevent the improper tracking of the patella through strength training for the glute minimus, medius and maximus. Be sure to include hip hitching and more advanced TFL strengthening including a leg swing to make it more running specific. Ankle proprioception and core strength make for a very well rounded protocol. I would start with the glute work and over time introduce the other exercises to avoid overloading the patient and losing compliance with the home exercise programme (HEP).

SSTM to the quads, working into the specific muscle groups that showed up as tight on assessment. I do not subscribe to the notion that VMO can be individually trained but that doesn't mean that inner range quads exercises are not part of the protocol (Inner range quad, page 181). Single leg squats performed with increasing depth over the weeks of rehabilitation, starting with minimal movement over a few centimetres depth at first, working slowly up to a 65-degree bend within a few weeks. Gain early control first then develop the range of motion alongside the attained abduction and glute max strength.

this injury is common in adolescents. Check over the good practice notes earlier in the book, designed to help those visiting a physio for the first time (page 26). How to prepare and what to wear can seem simple but many do not think about these aspects of attending therapy.

The physio will want to discuss where and when you first noticed the pain, how it developed and what your symptoms are today. The use of a pain scale can help to identify how bad the issue is and how much activity you can do before it starts to hurt, plus how quickly it settled down.

Testing will be in the form of functional testing, such as a single leg squat and checking strength around the hip and glute area to find out if you are losing support for the knee at the hip, whilst also assessing the foot and ankle to see if there is any underlying instability there.

In some cases you will require treatment as well as exercises, but in the main, this condition is well served by strengthening exercises. In those that are hypermobile, that is, they have more flexibility than most, then it can be effective to use massage to loosen off areas of tight muscle rather than to set stretches, as it is not desirable to lengthen the tendon and ligament when dealing with this problem. Targeting treatment to the muscle is a much better way of equalizing the length/tension relationship of the soft tissues.

GETTING BACK TO RUNNING

This is an issue that often affects the younger runner, so if you're in this demographic you shouldn't place any pressure on yourself. Hopefully with a long running career to look forward to, this is a great opportunity for you to correct any faulty biomechanics. Use your return to running to try out a training schedule that encompasses lots of strength and conditioning exercises that follow the self-treatment exercise goals and develop you

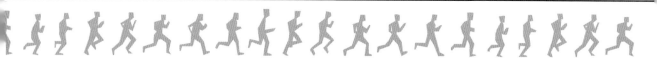

Sport has always been a big part of my life. I have competed in triathlon, swimming and cross country running since the age of eight and more recently started cyclocross. In my main sport, triathlon, I progressed to compete at national level and I am currently the fastest in the North East. In 2013 I caught glandular fever, which resulted in me having to stop swimming training for a couple of months and cycling and running training for just over a year, as these activities were too much of a drain on my energy levels. Once I was well enough to start training again, I only had a short amount of time until the North East Triathlon Talent Team selections. After such a long period out, I knew I had to work hard at the running and cycling if I was going to have a chance of being selected. However, I was soon devastated as within the first couple of weeks I was getting too much pain in my knees to train at either activity.

The pain was a continuous dull ache, but became a sharp and stabbing pain behind my knee cap as soon as I put any impact on my knees. Though I had experienced a similar pain in the past, it had never been as intense. I was extremely worried that this would affect my chances of team selection.

My mum booked an appointment for me to see Paul. Initially he examined my knees, posture and the strength of the muscles around my legs. He was able to diagnose the problem as Chondromalacia Patellae – my kneecaps were pointing slightly inwards, which was causing rubbing and the pain. I was given a number of strengthening exercises to complete daily initially, building up to twice a day, with increased reps. The exercises concentrated on the abductor muscles and gluteal, such as clams, squats and side leg raises, to try and pull my knees back into position. Paul also strapped my knees with sports tape to hold the kneecap in the correct position.

I had regular physio, which included sports massage and manipulation of the joint, and after two months the pain started to ease and I could finally start to train properly again. Within four months I was able to complete the 140-mile Coast to Coast bike ride in two days, staying in the saddle so as to not put too much pressure on my knees. Six months after starting treatment, I was selected as part of the team to represent the North East at the Nationals where I finished mid-field which I was very pleased with. Paul has advised that the Chondromalacia Patellae will come and go as my body grows and develops so I still continue with the strengthening exercises on a daily basis and wear the sports tape as a preventative measure.

even further. Running should be little and often, opting for fewer miles and more focus on technique than pre-injury. If you can get some expert help, consider choosing a forefoot strike over heel strike as this can offload the knee. Keep an eye on your discomfort levels at the knee. Don't run if your pain is increasing, but in the first instance you may have to accept a little soreness at a very low level as you return to running.

Meniscus cartilage injury

What is it?

The knee has a major articulation between the femur (thigh bone) and the tibia (shin bone). These two bones meet with surfaces that don't match up particularly well and so the joint congruency is improved with two horseshoe-shaped pieces of cartilage called the menisci. The menisci not only

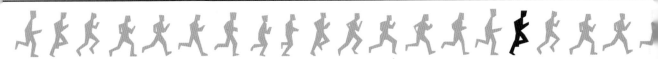

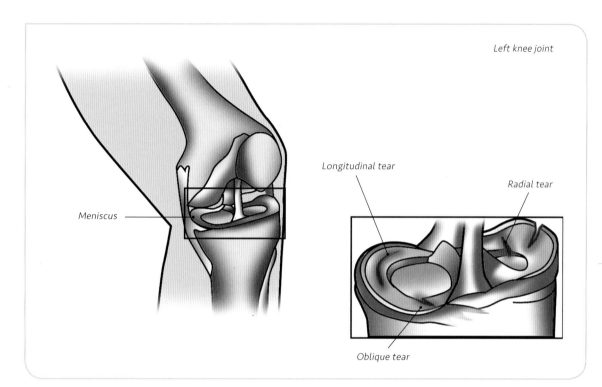

Meniscus

Longitudinal tear

Radial tear

Oblique tear

improve congruency of the joint, but act as shock absorbers during activity. These are fragile and with age become more susceptible to injury. The biomechanics of the knee joint play a huge part in the maintenance of the menisci, as a perfectly aligned knee will be much less likely to damage the cartilage. There is no evidence to support the notion that running alone speeds up the degradation of these structures or the knee itself, however, it is logical to accept that poor alignment will damage the surfaces and everything between at a faster rate.

Females have been shown to suffer cartilage injuries more than men, but I have to say that the evidence from my clinic shows a 50/50 split.

The cartilage can tear (acute injury) or break down (chronic injury) over time. The acute injuries usually occur with a twisting motion as the two bones provide both a compressive and rotational force to the cartilage. This is sufficient to cause a tear within the material, which can be in a variety of positions.

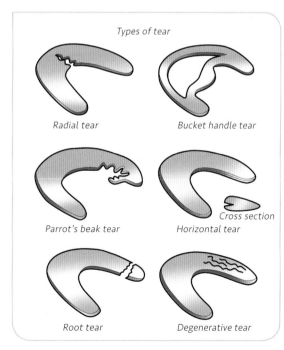

Types of tear

Radial tear

Bucket handle tear

Parrot's beak tear

Horizontal tear

Cross section

Root tear

Degenerative tear

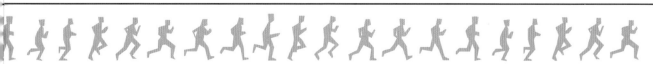

SELF-ASSESSMENT

There is a test, but if you have only slightly hurt your knee, this is quite a risky test as it may well hurt more afterwards.

Start by going through the mechanism of injury. Did you twist awkwardly, was there immediate pain and yet no obvious swelling for 7–12 hours? If this is the case and you have a knee that feels unstable, painful and may have felt like it locked for a short time, then it is highly likely that you have a cartilage injury.

If you want to check further, then – with caution – try duck walking. Squat down as far as you can go so your bottom is close to the floor, then without raising your bottom up, try walking forwards. Immediate pain in the affected knee or a total inability even to attempt the exercise is a positive test for a meniscus cartilage injury.

TREATMENT

I have seen people recover from the operation very quickly indeed and return to running and playing sport within six weeks. The issue still remains that if your menisci became worn down due to a chronic injury, then whilst an operation is one route on offer, physiotherapy is now arguably the leading treatment. There are bound to be some biomechanical issues that need sorting out ahead of a return to running and the knee itself needs to settle down. Many therapists will suggest that you give up running altogether; however, I take a more pragmatic approach. My aim is to get you pain-free, with great biomechanics through strength and condition exercise and orthotic inserts for your shoes. Once pain-free on walking we simply increase your strength functionally and a gradual return to running is achieved within your capabilities.

SELF-TREATMENT

The self-treatment can be seen as threefold: firstly avoid the injury through good prehab, secondly, pre-operatively; and thirdly, post-operative rehabilitation.

There is also the need for core strength. This is a common factor in so many cases for rehabilitation and for that matter injury prevention. Basic core strength exercises (Core muscles (strength), page 176, Swiss ball abduction in side plank, page 180,

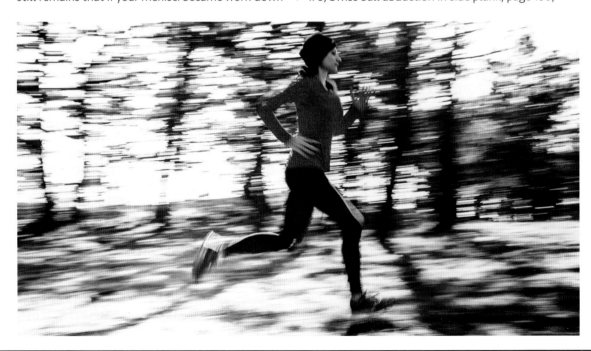

The current thinking is only to operate if the knee is locking, or the patient is in significant pain and is desperate for the surgery, as there just isn't sufficient evidence that surgery is providing enough benefit (Kruse, 2012).

This leaves us with the burden of responsibility to help those turned away from surgery. Strengthening exercises are key and from the exercise appendix, I suggest the following: Single leg balance, page 171, The clam – hip abduction/rotation (strength), page 173, Single leg squat (strength), page 175, performed as described in the ITB and PFPS section (see page 104), Glute activation (strength), page 175, Core muscles (strength), page 176, ITB Tensor fascia latae (stretch), page 178, Inner range quad, page 181. Eventually move onto Clock lunges, page 185 and Multi-direction hopping, page 186.

and Bridge, page 184) are vital for a good outcome. Here the core is integrated with the rehab: Single leg balance, page 171, The clam – hip abduction/rotation (strength), page 173, Hip adductors (stretch), page 174, Single leg squat (strength), page 175, Glute activation (strength), page 175, Core muscles (strength), page 176, Hamstring/core combination (strength), page 174, ITB Tensor fascia latae (stretch) page 178, Swiss ball abduction in side plank, page 180, Inner range quad, page 181 and Bridge, page 184.

WHAT TO EXPECT FROM A PHYSIOTHERAPIST

The testing can sometimes produce the same pain you have been experiencing as we search for the diagnosis. We try to keep it to a minimum but it is important that we achieve a robust diagnosis. The likely outcome is onward referral for an MRI scan though at the same time the physio can give you some good exercises to do that can both help with the alignment and also prepare you for surgery.

GETTING BACK TO RUNNING

This is dependent upon the extent and success of your surgery, or if you chose to take the non-surgical route, and of course how bad your injury is in the first place. In the event of surgery you will have two weeks with some stitches in or at least Steristrips over the small holes where the instruments entered your knee. Rehab can start immediately after you leave the hospital with some basic exercises such as the inner range quad, but as a runner you will be able to move quickly onto the continued development of your glute activation, core strength, and abduction/adduction strength.

Once you are pain-free when walking, if your consultant agrees then you can start with running-related exercises such as the squat, single leg squat and eventually hopping drills. The natural progression is onto running and some have made this transition in a few weeks.

There is a substantial risk of further pain, the development of osteoarthritis and further damage to your meniscus over time. Research has shown further damage to be a probability and not a certainty. You will read countless tales of people who have run several marathons since their surgery without issue. I would surmise that these individuals had minor surgery and started out with good alignment and that they suffered an acute injury rather than a chronic degradation of the cartilage prior to surgery. Every case is individual and every case needs a good medical examination and a structured, pain-free return to running.

THE KNEE

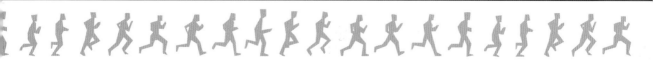

At the time I injured my knee I was running regularly, competing in a couple of marathons a year sandwiched by a few half marathons. Initially I'd started running about 12 years ago to lose some weight and get fit and had never had any real problems until this happened. I was training an average of three times a week around my job as I was working in a secure training centre for young offenders, which was a fairly active job anyway. One day, during a PE lesson, I joined in with the kids and was playing tennis against one of them. I remember going long for the ball and as I reached up and swiped for it I felt my left knee go. It wasn't nice. It felt as though something had crumbled except the accompanying noise was more of a sharp crack. Pain immediately seared down the side of my leg from my kneecap but I found I was still able to bear weight and limped about on it. It swelled and stiffened up shortly after and I proceeded to work through what felt like one of the longest shifts of my life as I felt it nag at me all day long.

After a few days the pain had subsided. I didn't want to risk running on it just in case I worsened the injury. I waited a full 10 days before I braved anything and chose to do a steady four-mile run, which I completed without any issues. Great I thought, but it was during the following weeks that I started to develop a niggling pain from the left of my kneecap down towards my calf. I pushed through it and even went out and bought a sturdy knee support, which seemed to do the trick. Every time that I stopped using the support the niggling pain would return. I knew I had to get it looked at by a professional.

I made an appointment to see my doctor. After explaining the symptoms to him he proceeded to prod and twist my troubled joint to test its flexibility and to narrow down which movements were causing me the most discomfort. Following

this he referred me for an orthopaedic appointment at the local hospital. After a few months of waiting for the appointment it came through and I was seen by the registrar. After explaining the problems I had she referred me for an MRI scan which, due to a convenient cancellation, I only had to wait two weeks to have.

Over the few months that this had been happening I had applied to take part in Operation Ultra, a competition held by Men's Running magazine. The prize was entry into an Ultra Marathon (in my case the LadyBower 50 in the UK), a load of free running gear, advice, treatment and training as well as being featured in the magazine itself. I was one of the lucky souls that were picked and it was through the magazine that I was referred to Physio&Therapy for a pre-training assessment. During this process Paul carried out a traffic light assessment on my legs to check their flexibility and generally what shape they were in. Here he flagged my knee as a problem that needed looking at and he also identified that I pronate when I run meaning my feet lean inwards when I step.

A month later I was back in the orthopaedic department looking at the results of my MRI scan. I had torn cartilage by over 1cm down the left-hand side of my kneecap and there was also a smaller tear down the right-hand side of the same knee. I was informed by the registrar that the best course of action to take in this scenario would be to have keyhole surgery. I asked whether it was safe to go ahead with the Ultra marathon and she agreed that I could as she didn't think my injury would worsen much by the time my operation was due. I agreed to it and was placed on the NHS waiting list.

I trained hard throughout the summer months; following my training plans closely that had been drawn up by the magazine. I was also monitored

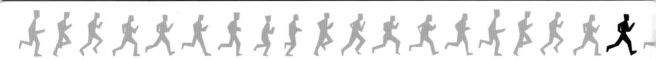

and offered strengthening exercises and advice by Paul whilst he administered sports massages for my aching legs.

In the meantime race day had crept up and was suddenly upon me. I commenced running at 7am and 11 hours later I finished running and was more than satisfied that I had completed my first ever Ultra-marathon. My knee held up throughout and fortunately was no hindrance.

The day of my operation arrived. I was prepped, anaesthetized and then operated on. After less than an hour in surgery I was returned to the ward in a very dozy state. The surgeon had performed a procedure called micro-fracturing in which a very small needle is repeatedly stabbed into the bone. The tiny holes automatically heal but during this process the fluid secreted from them also repaired my cartilage. A scar tissue would form covering the tears in the cartilage patching it together again. I was told that I would need crutches following the procedure for up to three weeks as I was not allowed to weight-bear until my knee healed enough to take the strain.

After two weeks of hobbling around on a set of crutches, the set became a single and after another week I was walking about comfortably unaided. Soon after this I attended my first physiotherapy appointment. To start with the treatment was extremely gentle and delicate. It consisted of a variety of very basic leg movements, lifting and holding at different angles both seated and standing. Each session lasted about 45 minutes and there were three sessions a week.

After a couple of weeks I was progressing well and was given a big red rubber band that would offer resistance to my exercises. As my strength grew I was able to progress to the next colour band, which was a tighter stretch and offered further resistance. After another couple of weeks my sessions were extended and following the initial raises and resistance sessions I spent a further 45 minutes taking part in what I can only describe as an indoor obstacle course of varying difficulty.

Exercises consisted of squats, seated balances, weaving in and out of bollards, and step-ups to name a few. Each week the obstacle course was set out differently and the exercises varied. I attended as many of the sessions each week as I could and following each session I felt the benefits and noticed my strength returning. After 10 weeks of this routine I was signed off the physiotherapy sessions and was deemed fit once again.

During my recovery time following the operation I had put on some extra weight due to my inactivity so I was more than eager to get out and run it off. I knew I had to take everything slowly and was prepared to start small. It was spring and I had eagerly signed up to do the Great North Run and the Loch Ness Marathon in September.

Starting back running after four months off wasn't easy. It was like I was starting from scratch just like I had 12 years previously. It was hard. I would run a mile or so then walk a bit, run another mile then walk some more. I'd do this until I was comfortable that my knee was going to take it and that I felt fit enough to start putting more distance in. Sure enough, after a month I was quickly working my way back to being on form and losing a chunk of the excess pounds I had gained.

Once again I spent my summer training, gently this time and by the end of it the Great North Run was upon me. I was feeling confident about it and managed to complete the race, narrowly missing out on my PB by 1½ minutes. I was happy with that. Later that month I took part in the Loch Ness Marathon, which I had done before but knew it would be more challenging this year. It was definitely a tough race but I did manage to complete it without any issues caused by my repaired knee. It reminded me that I could still go the distance.

I am now training for a further three marathons this year and am even considering taking part in another Ultra. I figure that as long as I'm careful I can keep on going. So that's what I do.

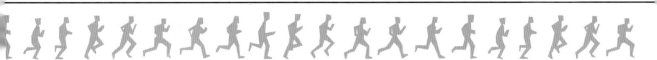

Pes anserinus bursitis

What is it?

Pain that is spontaneous and occurs in the medial aspect of the knee, just inferior to the patella (as pictured below).

The area is an attachment point of three muscles, namely the sartorius (knee and hip flexion, abduction and lateral rotation of hip), gracilis (hip adduction, medial rotation and flexion, plus some flexion of the knee as well) and semitendinosus (one of the hamstrings). The coming together of these three muscle tendons with all their many actions can cause a lot of friction for a runner, therefore irritating the little fluid-filled, sac, the bursa, which is designed to reduce friction at this attachment point.

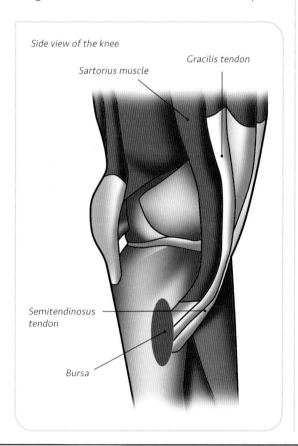

Side view of the knee

Gracilis tendon

Sartorius muscle

Semitendinosus tendon

Bursa

Runners will tend to get pain on the inside of the knee, similar to that of ITB friction syndrome, which is on the lateral aspect of the knee.

EARLY WARNING SIGNS

- Pain just medial and slightly lower than the kneecap
- Stiffness in the medial knee first thing in the morning
- Tension in the three key muscles
- Pain walking upstairs or uphill.

COMMON REASONS FOR INJURY

- This is primarily an overuse injury, which means you may have stepped up your training programme a little too fast
- Your running shoes may be nearing the end of their lifespan
- Muscle weakness, particularly in the hip area.

PROGRESSION OF THE INJURY

As the hamstrings start to tighten, runners can develop a snapping sensation on the inside of the knee. Swimming breaststroke can become painful (often referred to as Breaststroker's Knee) and you may well have sufficient inflammation to have pain at night.

It is worth reading the section on meniscal tears as often these two injuries present together.

SELF-ASSESSMENT

The pain is on the medial side of the shin just below the knee joint, where the adductors and the most medial of the hamstrings meet. Irritation here can be a common cause of knee pain and can be confused with a meniscus or MCL injury – so also perform the tests for these two injuries to rule them out.

Gently test the abductors by creating a stress over the medial knee (also tests the MCL). Push the inside of your foot into the floor to gently open the inside of the knee joint. Pain coming from just below the knee joint line and not in the middle of the joint line suggests pes anserinus rather than MCL. If you add some active knee flexion at the same time and pain increases, then it is further evidence of this injury and not MCL. Feeling along the length of the MCL ligament would not be painful, but touching the top of the tibia would be.

TREATMENT

Treatment is initially rest, to allow the tendons to settle, a reduction in the tension within the three key muscles (sartorius, gracilis and semitendinosus) through soft tissue massage, and where appropriate using deep transverse frictions (DTF). DTF is a sawing-like action of the fingertips or thumb over the injured tendon to stimulate the cell growth within the structure and encourage the healing process.

SELF-TREATMENT

Start with isometric contractions so there is no joint movement. This will rest the knee and reduce the likelihood of further irritation. Then start to build in some gentle movement with the same fundamental exercises, details below, and gradually make these more functional.

An example would be working on the adductors. Initially just squeeze a ball between your knees, then work up to squeezing the ball as you perform a squat. Eventually you can progress to Swiss ball abduction in side plank, p. 180 and Single leg squat (strength), p. 175, concentrating on alignment, therefore using the adductors as a stabilizer).

WHAT TO EXPECT FROM A PHYSIOTHERAPIST

When you see a physiotherapist, you should expect to undergo a full examination of the knee, foot mechanics and pelvic stability. The assessment is looking for either a biomechanical issue or overuse injury, so the physiotherapist will test for muscle length, strength and also joint movement and alignment.

The treatment will largely consist of soft tissue work and exercise prescription, but the cause of the injury must be addressed for you to have a full recovery, so expect plenty of functional testing and exercises to correct your biomechanics.

GETTING BACK TO RUNNING

Following a period of rest, you will move through your rehabilitation primarily doing static exercises, eventually you will be allowed back to running, short intervals at first.

Start off with rehabilitation runs of 3 minutes in duration x 5, stopping to perform Quads stretch, p. 182, Hip adductors (stretch), p. 174, and Hip flexors (stretch), p. 173 during the breaks. Rest for 2 days then try 5 x 4 minutes, rest for 2 days then increase the runs to 5 minutes long. Continue with this until 7-minute runs are possible, then start to reduce the set numbers as the time increases until you are running 3 x 10 minutes, then 2 x 15 min and 2 x 20 minutes. From here you can start to access your usual training programme again.

PRACTITIONER PROTOCOL

- Treat this as you would any bursitis, but soft tissue work to the gracilis, sartorius and semitendinosus is useful for recovery
- DTF to the insertion
- Shockwave therapy over the site of injury. 500 shocks at 10 per second using 1.5Htz, followed by 2000 shocks at 10 per seconds using 2.5Htz. 4 sessions 1 week apart
- Eccentric loading for the adductors and hamstring (Hamstring/core combination (strength), page 174 and Swiss ball abduction in side plank, page 180)
- Hip adductors (stretch), page 174.

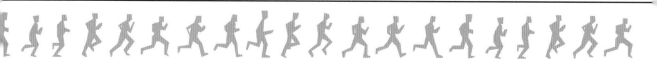

Osgood–Schlatter disease

What is it?

Osgood-Schlatter disease is a teenage problem, more common in boys rather than girls, and affects those who are running a lot (either through team sports or competitive running). The pain comes on just below the knee where the quadriceps tendon inserts into the tibia – the tibial tuberosity.

EARLY WARNING SIGNS

- Pain below the knee
- Swelling or bump appearing below the knee
- Sudden growth spurt with pain below the knee
- Tired and tight quadriceps muscles.

COMMON REASONS FOR INJURY

As a growing child, the long bones in the legs and arms increase, not uniformly along the length, but at two growth plates near to each end; rather like sticking a bit on at each end to increase the length. These growth plates are present until late teens/early twenties when they harden and you stop growing.

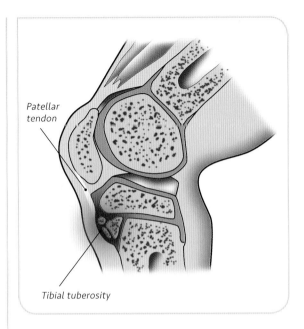

Patellar tendon

Tibial tuberosity

It is important to understand that these growth plates exist as they are a point of weakness for injury in the adolescent. In the case of Osgood-Schlatter, the growth plate is where the quads tendon attaches to the tibia.

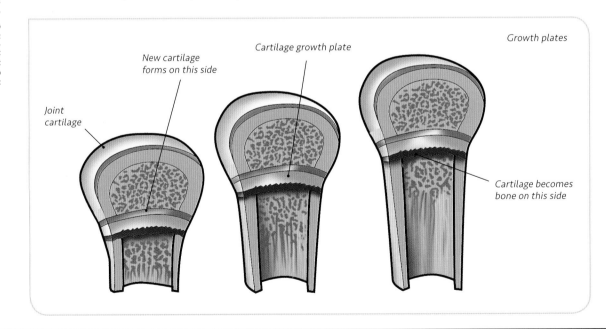

Joint cartilage

New cartilage forms on this side

Cartilage growth plate

Growth plates

Cartilage becomes bone on this side

PRACTITIONER PROTOCOL

Usually you are faced with a patient who is active and motivated to stay active. Saying the wrong thing at this stage can be fatal in terms of keeping the athlete connected to their sport. Encouragement is what's required above all else: keep them going to the club or track, to participate up to an agreed level of discomfort. I usually say 3/10 so it is low enough to keep the foolhardy from hurting themselves and high enough to allow them to at least complete the warm-up if that's possible.

As stretching can cause irritation to the insertion of the quads, I suggest regular massage, frequently teaching some of the basic techniques to the parents for daily input. Talk up the virtues of warming the muscle before activity and the use of the foam roller for self-treatment.

Try seeing this client every two or three weeks, and suggest they use a height chart at home to look for bursts in growth and therefore accommodate more physiotherapy at these times to keep the muscles as loose as possible.

Recommend gentle stretching, but only to the point of light pull, to try to keep a 'little and often' approach to gently maintaining some length in the quads.

Soft tissue should encompass trigger point therapy, fascia release and general effleurage. Release the TFL and strengthen the glutes to maintain balance within the knee and encourage general core strength and hamstring stretches.

It is the constant pull from tight quads (possibly due to an erratic growth battle between bone and soft tissues) that can irritate this growth plate and cause pain and inflammation, in the form of a visible, almost cartoon-like bump below the knee.

PROGRESSION OF THE INJURY

Osgood-Schlatter disease will continue to wax and wane dependent upon the load that is placed upon it, but I don't believe you can ask a sporty young adult to stop exercise altogether. I think with careful management within the parameters of moderate discomfort, sport should continue, albeit on a moderated basis. If the symptoms become too painful to continue, then periods of rest will be required, however, this disease typically dissipates over about two years.

SELF ASSESSMENT

Provided you are a teenager, this self-assessment will be relevant, however, if you are middle-aged, it is unlikely that you have a growth plate disorder so consider other knee injuries.

Feel just below your kneecap, for an area of obvious swelling. Compare this to the good knee, which should resemble a slightly raised area of bone, rather than a puffy circle of swelling. If this area is where you get most of your pain and is tender to touch, you may well have Osgood-Schlatter disease.

TREATMENT

Soft tissue treatment is key here and might just be one of the best applications of sports massage for any injury. Given the likelihood that stretching can exacerbate the problem owing to

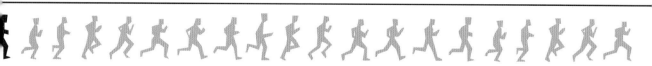

the pull on the injury site, the ability to soften and perhaps lengthen the muscle tissue in the quads without any pull at all is priceless. I have used soft tissue massage on patients to great effect and kept adolescent runners active and engaged with the sport throughout their period of injury.

SELF-TREATMENT

Gentle stretching of the quads; this does need to be gentle so as not to further irritate the insertion point. Instead of stretching you could use a foam roller, which causes less pull on the insertion.

The relevant exercises are Hip flexors (stretch), p. 173, Hamstrings (strength), p. 174, Glute activation (strength), p. 175, Core muscles (strength), p. 176 and Quads foam rolling, p. 181.

Daily massage, from a friend or parent is helpful, ask your physio to demonstrate some basic techniques.

WHAT TO EXPECT FROM A PHYSIOTHERAPIST

There is little that can be done for the young athlete except to keep the quads as loose as possible through the period of soreness, usually 18 months. Osgood-Schlatter disease is a self-limiting condition in that it will subside all on its own and in effect burns itself out. Sadly, some youngsters will lose their love for sport and the 18-month period is enough for them to find other pursuits and forget running altogether (or rugby or football).

GETTING BACK TO RUNNING

The best management strategy that I have employed successfully over the years is to instruct the patient to run or play at 80% effort as a maximum, to stop after 50% of their normal duration or when the pain becomes more noticeable and to use ice and rest to recover from bouts of exercise. This is largely an undesirable conversation to be having with a motivated teenager whose life revolves around running, but it's the best on offer.

Fat pad impingement/ Hoffa's fat pad

What is it?

The body several fat pads in key areas aimed at reducing impact, friction or for cushioning. The knee has a large fat pad as shown in the picture below.

This fat pad can become impinged, especially in those who have a greater propensity to over-extend their knee. Most of the injuries seen to the fat pad happen when someone has hyperextended in an acute way, through slipping on mud or ice or falling foul of a hole whilst out running. The most common injury is when the patella (kneecap) impinges on an inflamed fat pad through a compressive force, such as a hyperextension injury.

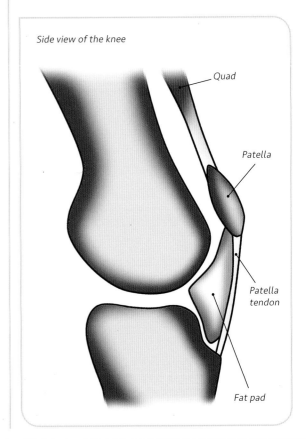

Side view of the knee

Quad

Patella

Patella tendon

Fat pad

EARLY WARNING SIGNS

- Excessive pain in the base of the knee joint anteriorly
- Pain on flexing or straightening the knee
- Suspect Hoffa's fat pad if your pain came on after direct impact or hyperextension injury.

COMMON REASONS FOR INJURY

- Hyperextension of the knee – such as kicking or slipping and the knee is forced backwards
- Increase in running training too quickly
- Impact to the kneecap.

PROGRESSION OF THE INJURY

If left untreated, the impingement will continue to aggravate the fat pad and pain will continue. If you were to try and run, the pain would build and build as the knee flexed and extended, pressure from running up inclines or stairs would be worse than flat running. With the correct treatment, the fat pad can settle and pain will be prevented quite quickly.

SELF-ASSESSMENT

The fat pad that lies tightly in the space just behind the lower portion of the kneecap can become irritated and inflamed, particularly after some hyperextension of the knee. Testing is difficult for someone to do themselves and even a physiotherapist would struggle to self-test this injury, though you may be able to rule out other conditions listed in this book to get this diagnosis.

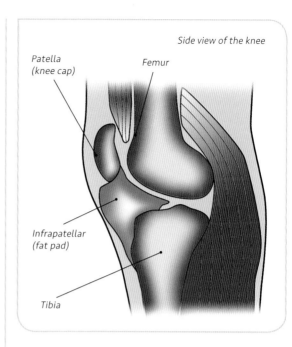

Side view of the knee

Patella (knee cap)

Femur

Infrapatellar (fat pad)

Tibia

PRACTITIONER PROTOCOL

- Use soft tissue to loosen the rectus femoris muscle tension
- Use kinesiology tape to lift the patella upward and also at the back of the knee, apply tape to a bent knee to provide a reminder not to hyper-extend the knee
- Advise on normal gait and rest from running, and ice until the pain has reduced to zero when walking
- Assess the hips, look for a reduction in movement on the affected side and assess for glute activation as well, there may be a functional issue higher up the chain that has led to this injury, which will need to be corrected. Whatever your thoughts on leg length inequality and symmetry, if the affected leg can be shown to be short, then the temporary use of a raise in that shoe can reduce hyperextension risk, although this requires careful assessment and sound clinical reasoning.

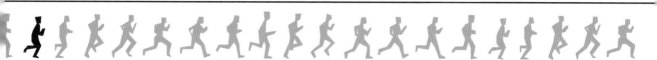

TREATMENT/SELF-TREATMENT

The treatment of choice initially is ice for 10 minutes every hour and taping down the top of the kneecap, so as to lift the bottom edge and create more space between the patella and the fat pad. Rest is indicated simply through the immediate pain on attempting to run and this can hang around for a long period if the runner decides to return too quickly.

Other treatments include anti-inflammatory medicines and surgery to remove enlarged fat pad tissue.

The relevant exercises are: The clam – hip abduction/rotation (strength), page 173, Hip flexors (stretch), page 173, Glute activation (strength), page 175, Core muscles (strength), page 176, Glutes (stretch), page 177, ITB Tensor fascia latae (stretch), page 178 and Inner range quad, page 181.

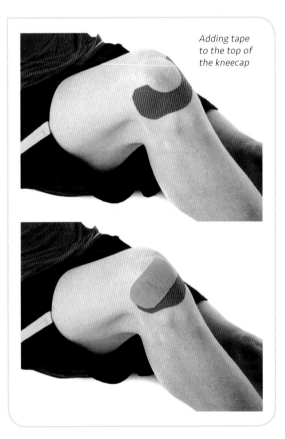

Adding tape to the top of the kneecap

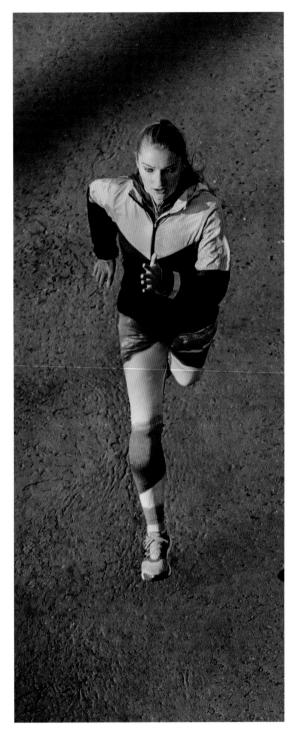

RUNNING FREE OF INJURIES

CLIENT STORY: TOM, 33

Having increased my running training quickly after a successful first marathon I developed a sharp pain in the lower part of my knee after I slipped when running in icy conditions. Pain continued when walking up or down stairs or when moving after sitting for long periods. The lower half of the knee was noticeably 'puffy' and sensitive. I took 3 days off running and spent a period stretching my quads and regularly icing the affected area. On return to running the pain and swelling instantly returned.

Having spent over 6 months unable to run whilst undergoing assessments via the NHS and unsuccessful treatment for patella tendonosis (including cortisone injections into the knee) I went to see Paul in desperation and worried my running career was finished less than 18 months after starting. Many of the symptoms had not changed significantly since the original injury and my knee was still slightly swollen and puffy. Paul undertook a new diagnosis involving testing pain levels on extension of the knee whilst holding the affected area and quickly diagnosed a possible Hoffa's syndrome likely brought on by a hyper extension of the knee when running on icy roads following a rapid increase in mileage, which had left my supporting muscles too fatigued to provide adequate stability.

Paul carried out deep tissue massage on my quads and surrounding muscles, looked closely at my hip stability and in particular my glute strength as they appeared to be under active on the left side following an ACL reconstruction 6 years previously. Paul used tape to lift the top half of my patella to reduce pressure on the fat pad and within 2 days much of the swelling that had been there for months had reduced significantly and I was walking downstairs with significantly reduced pain.

A combination of continued glute strengthening which included clam exercises, leg abductions and side stepping with a resistance band, massage into the quads and TFL and stretching for my hip flexors, I made a rapid return to running. I gradually eased back into running for short periods every 2-3 days and supported with cross training including aqua jogging. Six weeks after treatment I was back into full training and have not seen a return of this injury, and 4 years down the line am able to run in excess of 100 miles a week without issues.

I have maintained much of the glute conditioning and engagement work I learnt with Paul to ensure a better balance in my hips and to stabilize my running gait.

WHAT TO EXPECT FROM A PHYSIOTHERAPIST

Testing is simple, the physiotherapist will push their thumb and fingertips into the side of the patella tendon and take your knee from a bent position to straight. Pain on extension will be a positive finding for fat pad impingement.

GETTING BACK TO RUNNING

The prognosis is excellent once the fat pad has reduced in size as no damage has been caused unless the acute injury has also caused some damage to the bone surface or cartilage. Do not try to rush back too soon, as the inflammation can return quickly with a new stimulus and set you right back to the beginning. Taping has been shown to be effective, but some runners getting back into training whilst the knee is taped can forget one day and cause a new inflammation to occur, so it's important to remember to tape. Take advice on when to start back and when to stop using ice and tape. A series of simple tests at the physio clinic will suffice.

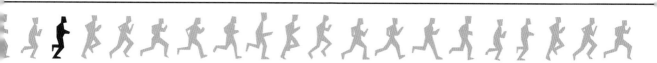

Medial Collateral Ligament (MCL) and Lateral Collateral Ligament (LCL)

What is it?

The ligaments either side of the knee joint are called the lateral collateral ligament (LCL) and the medial collateral ligament (MCL). These two ligaments protect against excessive movement of the knee joint medially or laterally. Injury to the MCL creates a greater degree of instability than any other ligament injury in the knee and must be fully healed before any sporting activity takes place to avoid future complications with the knee joint or surgery to any other injured part of the knee.

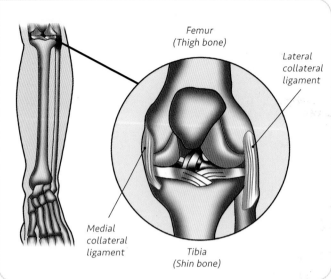

Femur (Thigh bone)

Lateral collateral ligament

Medial collateral ligament

Tibia (Shin bone)

The most common injury is the MCL and it occurs often in skiers or team sport players such as football or rugby. The MCL is an underrated supporting structure of the knee and its fibres not only run from above the knee joint to below it, but slip inside slightly and are continuous with the medial meniscus cartilage. When damaging the MCL it is not uncommon to damage the medial meniscus as well and also the anterior collateral cruciate ligament.

The LCL is less commonly injured. It is on the outside of the knee and passes between the femur (thigh bone) and the tibia (shin bone). It prevents the knee joint opening up at the lateral margin.

Any stress that is applied to the knee in either a lateral or medial motion (such as a sliding tackle from the side, stressing the LCL due to the medial movement of the lower leg) will have the potential to cause damage.

EARLY WARNING SIGNS

As a traumatic injury, this isn't an injury that can be seen coming on gradually. However, in an attempt to try and differentiate this from other knee pain, here is a basic list:

- Pain either side of the knee joint
- Medial pain is MCL, lateral pain is LCL
- Tenderness over the joint line when pressed
- Pain on gentle stress to the joint in the direction of the injured fibres.

COMMON REASONS FOR INJURY

This traumatic injury, where a stress has been placed on the ligaments, usually happens during such activities as football, rugby and skiing, however, a sudden fall during running, either through slipping off a kerb or sidewalk, twisting your ankle or slipping on ice can be enough to cause injury to these knee ligaments.

PROGRESSION OF INJURY

Damage to a ligament as discussed in relation to the ligaments of the foot (see page 61), can be graded in three ways. Grade 1 is the least injury involving only just a few of the fibres of the ligament and is usually just a sprain of the fibres, grade 2 is where the sprain involves a partial rupture of the ligament, and grade 3 is a total rupture.

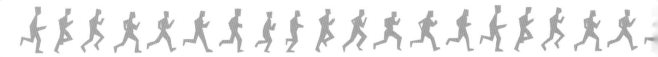

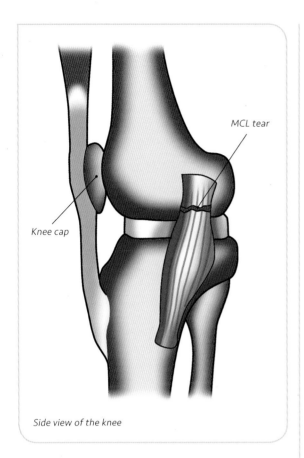

Side view of the knee

SELF-ASSESSMENT

The pain will be over your medial knee joint line. Feel for this by using your fingertips around the medial knee and gently flex your knee back and forth to feel for the joint moving. The MCL stretches just above the joint and inserts just below, so pain all along this line can suggest this injury.

Test the theory by creating a stress over the ligament (gently though). Push the inside of your foot into the floor so as to gently open the inside of the knee joint. Immediate pain should confirm some damage to this area.

TREATMENT

When dealing with a grade 1, the best policy is rest and the use of tape to support the ligament against any further damage. Usually four weeks would be enough including a gradual return to running, albeit with the strapping still present until six weeks after the injury.

Grade 2 would require a full brace, to ensure that no further damage was caused and to afford the fibres time to heal over the full six to eight weeks. A gradual and measured return to running would be required alongside some strengthening similar to that for knee tracking problems. This will ensure good control about the knee from higher up the chain and therefore reduced stress on the ligament.

A grade 3 full rupture will take six to eight weeks to heal and this is just the beginning of the journey back to running again. Slow build-up is required so as not to stress the ligament with a now deconditioned kinetic chain. If managed correctly, there shouldn't be any real long-term implications so long as no other damage has been caused requiring surgical intervention (for example the ACL or menisci being torn as well).

Treatments will include deep transverse frictions to the ligament once it has ended the acute phase. I have used shockwave therapy to great effect on these injuries speeding up the healing process and delivering a faster return to play.

SELF-TREATMENT

There is little to say about self-treatment when the main focus is on rest, however, you can ensure that you are cross training and working on key aspects of functional training to make you a stronger, more resilient athlete on your return from injury. Therefore, the exercises to be followed are Towel grabbing (strength), page 167, Tibialis posterior (strength), page 170, Peroneals–ankle eversion (strength), page 170, The clam – hip abduction/rotation (strength), page 173, Glute activation (strength), page 175 and Core muscles (strength), page 176.

WHAT TO EXPECT FROM A PHYSIOTHERAPIST

You should definitely attend to see a physiotherapist for formal diagnosis and advice on what sort of

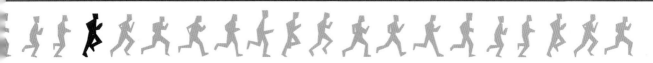

brace to use. There are some great treatment strategies available for the surrounding tissues and directed at the injured ligament itself. Assessment can be a little painful as we need to stress the fibres slightly to ascertain the grade of the injury, in extreme cases we may need a scan. One of the key issues for the physiotherapist is to see if anything else has been damaged, as it is not uncommon for the meniscus cartilage and anterior cruciate ligament to be injured at the same time as the medial collateral ligament.

GETTING BACK TO RUNNING

Definitely no running for the six weeks it takes for the ligament to heal, and even then proceed with absolute caution. Whilst the soft tissues have healed in this time, they are vulnerable. It is highly likely that you will be fine to start some slow and short jogging at the six-week point, however, change of direction and sideways type movements are to be totally avoided. In short, it's not OK to go back to 5-a-side football at the same time as you can jog to the end of the road and back.

CLIENT STORY: TOM, 23

I am a keen runner and also play football for a local team, which involves training twice a week and matches at the weekend. I tend to run more in the off-season as I don't have time to fit in as much as I would like between games.

I picked up my injury on the back of putting my knee through too much. I'd been running a lot more recently and playing numerous games of football each week as well and had started to feel discomfort in my knee. I went in for a tackle during a match, which wasn't particularly strong and didn't involve direct force from an opponent. As the tackle occurred I felt more severe pain in my knee than I had done previously. Not only did it prevent me from being able to run, it was a real struggle to walk, with shooting pain down the outside of my knee as the joint flexed and extended.

Paul was recommended to me by one of the other players and he referred me for an MRI scan, which confirmed that the Medial Collateral Ligament had torn in my right knee. As well as this I had fluid on the joint and had chipped my femur, though these were side issues to the main problem with the ligament. From here the plan was put together, to get me back to the ultimate goal of playing football again. The first part of this was wearing a knee brace for six weeks, which worked to get the ligament healing initiated.

Once I was done with the knee brace, the re-strengthening began. This involved seeing Paul once a week to have direct work done on the knee and surrounding areas, while I was also given various exercises designed to gradually re-strengthen the knee. After a couple of months of a programme that got more strenuous every week, I got myself out running and before long I was doing some sport-specific drills ahead of getting back in to football training. This provided a slight setback in that whenever I used the outside of my foot to kick the ball I could still feel pain in my knee. On the back of this, the rehabilitation plan was altered to cater for the delayed improvement. Eventually, having worked closely with Paul, I found myself back in training, and a bit further down the line back playing football.

I returned to playing football around 20 months ago, and all appears to be well with my knee. I still play two games a weekend and every now and then another game in the week. Without the detailed rehabilitation plan put together, from the knee brace to getting back into training, I believe that I'd still be having problems as a result of not approaching the injury correctly. I continue to enjoy football and running and owe all this to the professional diagnosis and rehabilitation.

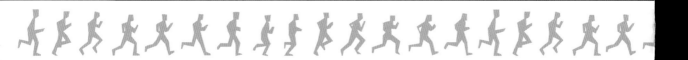

Once you have graded the injury and it is clear the patient is past the critical 72 hours post-injury, then adductor massage and DTF to the MCL work very well.

Depending upon the severity of the lesion, you may need to brace the knee with a structural knee support for six weeks, these are fairly inexpensive at around £35/$50 for a cheap one, but the support must have a hard material of some sort along the medial edge to prevent any valgus knee movement and be able to set the knee extension to minus 5 or 10 degrees to avoid straightening.

Treatment after this has repaired will be to restore knee extension and functional strength. Weekly treatment sessions have proven very effective for a speedy return to running.

Anterior Cruciate Ligament (ACL) and Posterior Collateral Ligament (PCL)

What is it?

The anterior cruciate ligament (ACL) and posterior collateral ligament (PCL) reside inside the knee joint itself and resist anterior or posterior glide of the femur on the tibia.

The ACL is the more likely to be injured and yet it is most unlikely to see either of these injuries caused purely by running. These ligaments tend to require a fairly significant trauma to rupture, however, their inclusion within the book is due to the vast number of runners taking part in other sports alongside their running.

In fact, it is quite rare these days to find someone who simply just runs. The allure of the weekly 5-a-side soccer game, or weekend netball session is extremely strong, even to the sub elite runner. The truly elite runners are unlikely to risk injury with other sports, but whilst there is a mild risk of, for example, an ACL rupture, the benefits of the challenging cutting and twisting

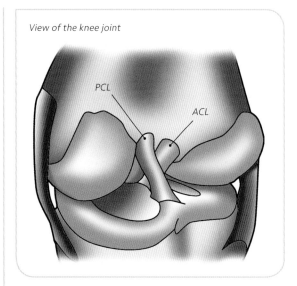

View of the knee joint

PCL

ACL

type movements on overall conditioning are also great.

PCL injuries occur in basically the same way, but with an alternate movement. So ACL injuries usually occur following deceleration with a direction change causing rotation about the knee; and the PCL will be damaged in the same way. Sudden stopping, twisting or turning or hyperextension of the knee can all cause the knee to give way and potentially damage any of the ligaments.

EARLY WARNING SIGNS

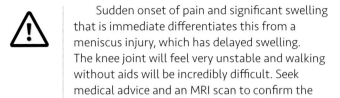

- Immediate swelling
- Intense pain
- Unable to load the knee at all
- Unable to walk.

COMMON REASONS FOR INJURY

This injury is most common following knee flexion during deceleration with rotation, so in short a change in direction at speed. This makes it very common in football, rugby and of course skiing.

If you do take a fall whilst out running or come off second in a sportsman's embrace on the rugby field, then sudden and immense pain with immediate swelling in the knee would be a fairly good clue that you have injured a cruciate ligament.

SELF-ASSESSMENT

This is an acute injury, whereby you will know the time, date and location of the injury. It will have involved some sort of twisting and deceleration activity with sudden pain and swelling.

Sudden onset of pain and significant swelling that is immediate differentiates this from a meniscus injury, which has delayed swelling. The knee joint will feel very unstable and walking without aids will be incredibly difficult. Seek medical advice and an MRI scan to confirm the diagnosis. Early intervention with surgery has the best outcome.

TREATMENT

Treatment for this injury is surgery. The best surgery is quick surgery, so you do not damage anything else. However, during the injury you are very likely to have also injured your MCL and medial meniscus cartilage. It is unlikely that you will get a good surgeon to operate until the MCL has healed, which will mean a period of time with a hinged knee brace on, unable to fully straighten your knee or bend past 90 degrees for a period of six to eight weeks.

Surgery requires a graft to be taken from the patella tendon or the hamstring tendon. The surgeon creates a new ligament from this graft and secures it in place through drilled holes with a screw

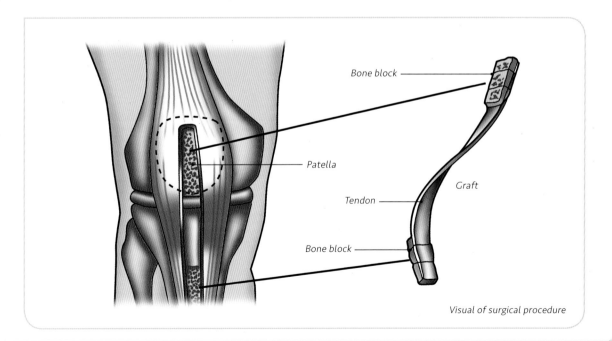

Bone block

Patella

Tendon

Graft

Bone block

Visual of surgical procedure

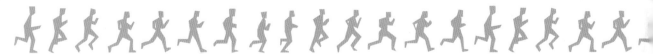

(in the case of the hamstring graft) or using the small lump of bone still attached to your graft (taken during the patella tendon graft procedure) as a natural end piece that cannot slip through the drill hole.

The rehab is slow, frustrating and long. Six months is the quickest return to full mobility, nine months is more typical and a year is considered the maximum required time.

ACL reconstruction post-surgery rehabilitation will depend on the surgeon's operative approach, but as a broad catch-all the following is a typical timeline for a standard rehabilitation programme (Kruse *et al.*, 2012; Hiemstra *et al.*, 2007).

- 0–2 weeks: minimize swelling and achieve full knee extension
- 2–6 weeks: Walking with normal gait, strengthening exercise progression
- 6–12 weeks: straight line jog – also swim, bike, cross trainer
- 3–6 months: Back to running – straight line, drills to include direction change
- 6–12 months: return to competitive sport.

Accelerated ACL Rehab (Kruse *et al.*, 2012; Hiemstra *et al.*, 2007)

0-2 WEEKS

- Protected full weight bearing
- Passive knee extension
- Range of movement exercise without restriction
- Static quadriceps contractions.

2-4 WEEKS

- Stationary bike
- Mobilize joints of knee
- Walking.

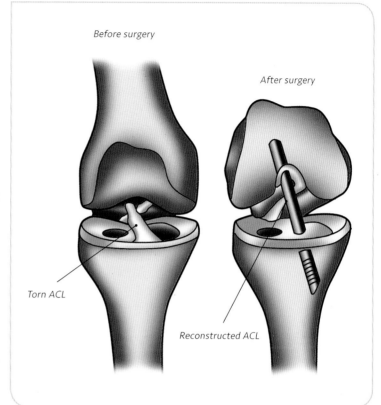

Before surgery

After surgery

Torn ACL

Reconstructed ACL

4-8 WEEKS

- Closed chain exercises
- Hamstring isometric and eccentric strengthening
- Hip strengthening.

8-12 WEEKS

- Progressive hamstring strength
- Quadriceps open chain 30 degrees extension block
- Swimming – front crawl leg kick only
- Outdoor bike.

12-16 WEEKS

- No extension block
- Return to running.

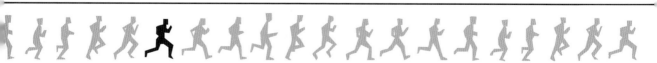

LESS THAN 20 WEEKS – RETURN TO SPORT PROVIDED
- No swelling during/after training
- Full range of movement
- Normal quads and hams function
- Excellent proprioception
- 100% confidence in stability of knee.

Once your operated-on knee has healed, you are actually equally as likely to injure your 'good' knee. Some people, including professional footballers, find that they never fully attain the level they were at prior to the injury. It's important therefore to stick with physio after your operation.

SELF-TREATMENT
Use the following exercises: Single leg balance, page 171, The clam – hip abduction/rotation (strength), page 173, Hip adductors (stretch), page 174, Hamstrings (strength), page 174, Single leg squat (strength), page 175, Core muscles (strength), page 176, ITB Tensor fascia latae (stretch), page 178 and Inner range quad, page 181.

WHAT TO EXPECT FROM A PHYSIOTHERAPIST
A physiotherapist would perform a drawer test to check for laxity, by pulling your tibia forwards on a bent knee. A comparison between the uninjured and injured side is a must as some of you will have old strains to the ligament or simply be very mobile through a great many of your ligaments.

Usually, you know immediately that you have done something serious and for the self-diagnosers out there, watch for the early swelling, as if you recall from the section on meniscus cartilage (see page 118), the swelling there comes 7–12 hours later.

Sadly, rehab is lengthy following reconstruction surgery. There are people who have soldiered on without a surgical repair (I for one did this for a time) but the risks of an unstable knee causing more damage to the cartilage and surrounding structures such as MCL or LCL are too great and I would suggest that you go under the knife as soon as possible.

GETTING BACK TO RUNNING
Getting back to running is relative quick compared to getting back to playing sport in open-field situations. The accelerated protocol (six months rehab) and the standard (9–12 months rehab) have straight-line running back in the programme at 8 and 12 weeks respectively.

PRACTITIONER PROTOCOL

Diagnosis and onward referral are the best options for early management. If you have an option for private MRI referral, then I suggest offering this to the patient if they want to proceed immediately without waiting to be seen. The average cost is between £200-300 in the UK at the moment and a serious runner will want to get on with the process. Failing that, a letter to the GP with a clear diagnosis and test results will help the process along.

In the meantime, recommend the following pre-operative exercises to help prepare for muscle wastage from inhibition and post surgery: The clam – hip abduction/rotation (strength), page 173, Hamstrings (strength), page 174, Glute activation (strength), page 175, Hamstring (stretch), page 178, ITB Tensor fascia latae (stretch), page 178, Inner range quad, page 181 and Bridge, page 184.

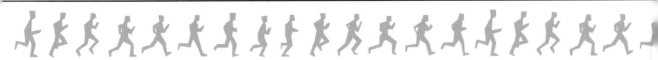

I injured my ACL in 2004 age 33 whilst playing football, which is not something I usually do as a runner. It was one of those quick moments where there was a impromptu ball found and everyone started by just kicking it between a crowd, but very quickly it became a full 'jumpers for goal posts' game. A sudden twist to move past an opponent and I dropped to the ground in unimaginable agony. Within seconds my knee was swelling and I couldn't walk at all, the pain was incredible but seemed to subside quite quickly unlike the swelling. That night I didn't sleep very well, despite ice and pain relief, I was unable to get comfortable, its strange to say, but I just inherently knew I had sustained a bad injury and wouldn't be back to running for a long time.

I had private medical insurance at the time so was seen almost immediately and within seconds found out I had ruptured my anterior cruciate ligament (ACL) and was therefore looking at 9-12 months rehabilitation. Interestingly however I was told that I could be back to some form of running much sooner than that, however I would require surgery. I had to wait a few weeks for the swelling to go down and the medial collateral ligament to heal, but it seemed to me that I was on the operating table pretty quickly after the injury.

I had a piece of my hamstring tendon taken and used to make a new ACL, complete with screws and staples. I left the hospital on pain medication and crutches along with a large brace from mid shin to mid thigh. Six weeks later I was free of the brace, crutches and thankfully all the medication.

It was very early on that I was on a stationary bike and I seemed to be doing basic exercises from day 1.

Being a keen runner, I was filling my usual training time with the exercises, perhaps doing too many of them in hindsight, but I wanted more than anything to get back running. Each visit to the physiotherapist seemed like a motivational high, I was being measured each time and assessed for function and clearly making excellent progress, often ahead of the normal time line. The words 'you can't speed bone healing' rang true at the end of every visit but I could optimize my recovery.

I was back running (of sorts) bang on 12 weeks, but it was painful. I didn't run for long and felt sure I was capable, but I felt incredibly down after that first jog, why was it still painful? I don't know what I expected, but after that first run I lacked motivation to try again and my attention to the exercises wavered for a week or so. I picked myself back up after a disappointing physio visit and got back to the programme, starting to run again a week later and with less pain. I remember running an interrupted mile for the first time around the 4 month marker and it seemed to mushroom from there, getting stronger and faster from there.

If I had one piece of advice for anyone out there reading this having just injured themselves with an ACL rupture, would be to get your head around the rehab as quickly as possible, be committed, obsessed even, but don't rush back to running, try to avoid the motivation blip that I encountered, and get yourself a great physio. I travelled to see Paul and his team and would do the same again.

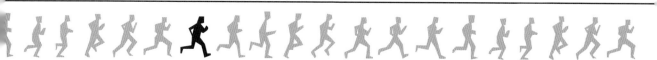

CHAPTER 5

THE HIP AND PELVIS

This section will include common running injuries that are above the knee up to and including the hip and pelvis.

Before moving any further up the body it is important to make reference to the pelvic bones and to better understand the anatomy, if only for the origins and insertions of the muscles that attach here and to understand the potential for movement and therefore biomechanical dysfunction, which can lead to a whole host of lower limb injury as a result of running.

Some myths about the pelvis need to be dispelled before we proceed. Whilst I am huge fan of Pilates, the analogy sometimes used by Pilates instructors of the pelvis being a water filled bucket the contents of which you have to work hard to maintain is not useful to aid our understanding of the anatomy (although it is helpful for postural alignment). This has led to many clients considering it as a whole unit, a rigid concave structure that is either tilted anteriorly (forward), level, or tilted posteriorly (backward). The fact is, the pelvis is two separate bones (innominate bones, each made up of the ilium, ischium and pubis) which are as complex in form as any bone in the body, with flat bony sections, sections with cutouts and a variety of knobbly landmarks.

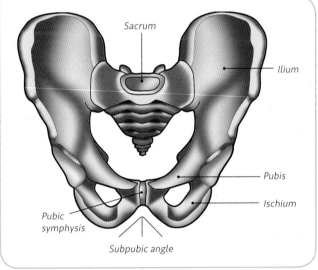

Sacrum

Ilium

Pubis

Ischium

Pubic symphysis

Subpubic angle

The two large bones that make up the pelvis are called the innominate bones. These two large, irregular shaped bones (that look a little bit like a human ear) are separated by a small piece of fibrocartilage between the two ischia (bones that are part of the pelvis) called the pubic symphysis at the very front and the sacrum bone at the posterior.

This means that the two innominate bones have a degree of freedom of movement. However, there is significant debate amongst practitioners about

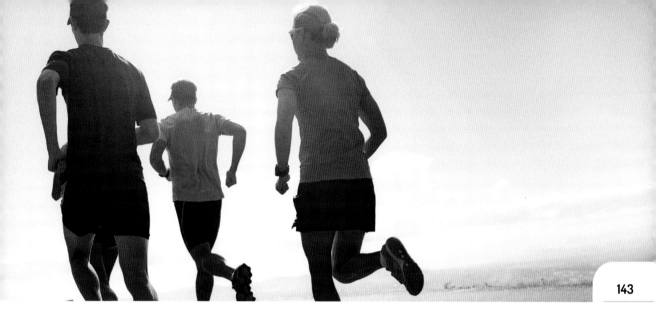

whether there is any available movement about the joint called the sacroiliac joint (SIJ) (Vleeming *et al.*, 2012). The notion fell out of favour with clinicians in the mid-20th century, though more recent scientific research now supports the idea of two degrees of motion in the three planes of movement of this joint. The clinical significance of this is yet to be made apparent, however, there are a great many practitioners with a wealth of experience who have applied therapeutic adjustment to the pressures within this joint, with a seemingly dramatic effect upon the patient's pain and mobility. The debate will rage on, but the answer will for now have to lie with your chosen practitioner, the treatments they use on you and the results you get from those treatments.

Dysfunction at the pelvis can result in tension to a vast array of muscles and potential injury, from the attachments of hamstrings, the adductors, quadriceps, hip flexors and the muscles that make up trunk and spinal stabilizers relevant to low back pain.

This section therefore includes:

- Quadriceps delayed onset of muscle soreness (DOMS)
- Trochanteric bursitis
- Groin or adductor strain
- High hamstring tendinopathy
- Piriformis syndrome
- Iliopsoas bursitis (anterior hip pain)
- Low back pain.

Quadriceps Delayed Onset Muscle Soreness (DOMS)

What is it?

The quadriceps (quads) tend not to give too much trouble when running, however, many runners complain of pain in this area after a long run as they struggle to go downstairs in the morning due to pain in the thigh (Tojima and Noma, 2015; Torres *et al.*, 2012).

The quads are essentially knee extensors, e.g. the muscles that straighten the bent knee. They are made up of four muscles (hence the name quad): vastus lateralis (the lateral quad), vastus medialis (the medial quad), vastus intermedialis (the deep quad) and rectus femoris, the central quad. Rectus femoris (Rec-fem) is the only quad muscle to cross the hip joint as well as the knee joint and as such is also a hip flexor as well as knee extensor.

The muscle injury here is minimal and not deemed a common running injury, but it has its place

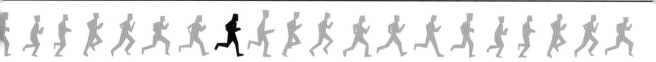

here owing to delayed onset of muscle soreness (DOMS) after long runs.

DOMS is a deep pain felt after the muscle has been worked beyond its usual threshold. It is painful to use the muscle at all and yet this generally abates after a few days, getting better with every passing moment and with gentle stretching and movement (Tojima and Noma, 2015, Torres et al., 2012).

COMMON REASONS FOR INJURY

DOMS occurs when you use the muscles in question more than they are used to. Heavy gym sessions and marathon or half marathon races are usually the cause, even for the most experienced athletes. However, a slight break from training and even a 10–15 minute run can cause muscle soreness in the days to come.

DOMS is often worst the morning after the morning after! That is, the delay is usually over 24 hours before the soreness reaches its peak.

PROGRESSION OF INJURY

The belief is that the muscle breaks down through overexertion and it's the damage that not only causes the pain, but also precedes the resultant strengthening of the unit. The muscle action that creates DOMS is the eccentric as opposed to concentric or isometric (Torres et al., 2012). Eccentric muscle contraction occurs as the muscle is lengthening. Think of your quads working eccentrically when you sit down, contracting to slow your descent and stop you hitting the chair with a bang. When running the quads are working to prevent your heel hitting your backside every time the hamstrings work to bend the knee. They work eccentrically on contact with the ground to moderate the impact and more so when running downhill.

This repeated contraction and then relaxation of the muscle fibres during the running action is how we move forward, each muscle working in unison with the others to create the desired movement, whilst other muscles are busy controlling unwanted movement. Think of the knee movement: as the quads straighten the knee, the hamstrings are slowly releasing the knee to moderate movement.

In addition, the adductors and abductors are working to prevent any movement to the sides, to keep the thigh in a straight forward path and not pulled out to the side or towards the midline. All this occurs without thought from us, but it's necessary for every step of the way. If the marathon takes between 30,000–50,000 steps, imagine all the individual muscle contractions that take place over the length of the race and you can see how some muscles could become more overloaded than others resulting in DOMS.

SELF-ASSESSMENT

Muscle soreness doesn't really have a self-assessment test; you will know that you exercised heavily the day before and have awoken to significant muscle stiffness and discomfort. Walking downstairs will be agony, but once you get moving the pain will subside a little.

TREATMENT

Many people suggest trying to go for a gentle jog, however there isn't enough scientific evidence to confirm an amelioration. Muscle stimulation (those machines that put electric impulses through your muscle and make them contract without you moving them) and massage have been shown to have better results. A swim is probably the least painful of all of these treatments.

SELF-TREATMENT

The quads are often stretched in a singular plane, pulling the foot up to the glutes and holding for a set period. The quads muscle group requires a full set of multi-position stretches: Hip flexors (stretch), page 173 and Quads stretch, page 182.

WHAT TO EXPECT FROM A PHYSIOTHERAPIST

There is little evidence that anything can be done for DOMS, however, massage has ranked higher in scientific research over light recovery exercise, electronic muscle stimulation or ice therapy (Torres et al., 2012) so a physio may recommend this.

RUNNING FREE OF INJURIES

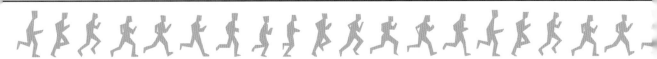

PRACTITIONER PROTOCOL

Not a usual reason for a patient to present to clinic, however, we often see clients post-marathon and so helping them return to training through recovery strategies is often part of our role as a practitioner.

Soft tissue massage, even electrostimulation of the muscles can help recovery. I usually suggest little and often in terms of exercise, and swimming is a great way to get the muscles moving without excess strain being placed on the already fatigued quads (there aren't any downhill sections in a pool).

GETTING BACK INTO RUNNING

If you have just run your first marathon, then give yourself some time out. A few days rest will work wonders, but keep moving little and often to keep the blood flow through the legs. The DOMS will ease slowly over a few days, but regular walking will help.

If you have DOMS because of new or more challenging training, then perhaps review whether what you are doing is too great a jump for you at this present time. Getting back to running will depend upon your ability to fight through the first few minutes of pain. Once moving you will find things feel so much better, but at this acute phase, little and often is the best route to regaining full pain-free function from your legs.

Trochanteric bursitis

What is it?

A bursa is a fluid filled sac found at most sites around the body where friction can occur. The sac is filled with synovial fluid and when irritated through a build-up of friction due to tight muscle/tendon units, the bursa inflames and pain is both local and at times referred. The previously slippery and smooth bursa is now enlarged, thickened and gritty, occupying an increased space and no longer providing

the smooth surface for the reduction of friction in the area. Pain is the overwhelming symptom and irritation is present with almost all movements of the area.

EARLY WARNING SIGNS

- Pain over the lateral upper thigh
- Pain particularly on movement
- Pain can start to radiate down the leg.

PROGRESSION OF THE INJURY

The pain will be mild at first but can progress very quickly indeed. The pain is located directly over the

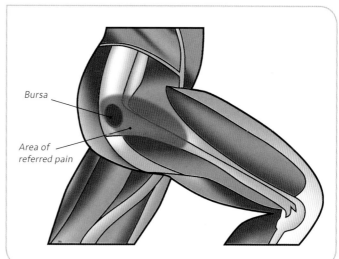

Bursa

Area of referred pain

greater trochanter, which is the bony bit you can feel on the outside of the top of your leg (often incorrectly referred to as the hip). The inflammation which initially only caused mild discomfort during a run will cause you pain when any movement causes rubbing over the area. You will be unable to run and walking will be painful.

SELF-ASSESSMENT

Pain and tenderness on the lateral hip and side flexion away from the affected hip may also produce the pain to help diagnose this injury.

TREATMENT

Most of the treatment needs to be in the release of the tissues that are causing the friction as well as reducing the swelling. Ice and anti-inflammatories are great at reducing pain and inflammation, whilst massage and trigger point therapy work well to reduce the tension in the ITB, abductors and hip rotators.

The treatment and management of trochanteric bursitis has shown non-operative treatments such as physiotherapy to help in the majority of cases and to be more effective than surgery or injection. There is also good evidence to support shockwave therapy

as an alternative treatment for this condition (Lustenberger *et al.*, 2013).

SELF-TREATMENT

Perform the following exercises: The clam – hip abduction/rotation (strength), page 173, Glute activation (strength), page 175, Hamstring/core combination (strength), page 177, ITB Tensor fascia latae (stretch), page 178, Sciatic nerve flossing, page 180, Quads foam rolling, page 181 and Quads stretch, page 182.

WHAT TO EXPECT FROM A PHYSIOTHERAPIST

This is one of those scenarios where the physiotherapist may have to prescribe some rest. You need the friction to stop in order to reduce the inflammation. The aim of treatment is to get the bursa to decrease in size and irritability.

Shockwave therapy has been shown to be very effective (Lustenberger *et al.*, 2013) and I have been using it as the first line of treatment alongside the corrective exercise therapy, with incredibly quick results. It is vital to reduce tension in the area, and so a physio will therefore work on the ITB release, abduction and core strength.

PRACTITIONER PROTOCOL

An injection can be very useful for the quick reduction of symptoms. However, consider what is the underlying cause of the pain? A full biomechanics review is needed. The pain usually comes on gradually over time and assessment is muddled with some passive and some active tests eliciting pain, but not all. Use the information you have from these tests alongside your hip and pelvis assessment to make an informed judgment on the cause.

If in doubt, strengthen what is weak and lengthen what is loose, but always check the pelvic alignment and the tension in the TFL and glute medius/minumus.

Useful exercises from the list in appendix 1 are: Single leg balance, page 171, The clam – hip abduction/rotation (strength), page 173, Hip adductors (stretch), page 174, Glute activation (strength), page 175, Core muscles (strength), page 176, Glutes (stretch), page 177, Quads stretch, page 182 and Piriformis stretch, page 183.

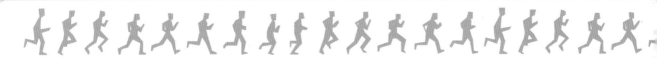

I have been a keen runner my whole life and its fair to say I have suffered at the hands of injury for a great deal of that time. Like most, I picked up the usual suspects early on, such as shin splints, knee pain and the like, but through some research and self help techniques I managed to muddle through some of those on my own with varying degrees of success. It was only when I started to turn to massage therapists and then physiotherapy that I really started to learn how to cope with my body, which I must confess is not your typical runner's physique. What I have learned thus far is, any weakness, any tightness or any area of fatigue is enough to deliver a fairly significant running injury. Therefore I have a set of exercises that I do every morning, comprising of the long list of exercises I have amassed over the years for my various ailments.

The most recent of these injuries was a new one for me, hip pain that seemed to travel down my leg a little. I did wonder if it was a trapped nerve in my back at first, but a visit to see Paul revealed this was the work of a small fluid filled sack aimed at reducing friction between my tendons and my bones. When working well, these sacks are thin and likened by Paul, to a double layer of plastic bag with oil between the layers, basically causing negative friction. However, once irritated they blow up like a puffer fish, reducing the space in the area and causing pain on movement and also at rest due to the inflammation present.

The fix for this issue is threefold: reduce the inflammation through ice, anti-inflammatory medication and rest; reduce the tension through soft tissue release; and finally strengthen the area to reduce the biomechanical fault.

I am pleased to say that I followed the advice and did my time in terms of rest and exercises and after a short period was able to start my running again. For someone like me, the information about the injury is as important as the knowledge on how to fix it. I like to understand and rather than being blasted with medical jargon, my brain likes the analogy of plastic bags and puffer fish, it helps me to understand what it is that I need to do so I can successfully fulfill my role in the process.

GETTING BACK TO RUNNING

This has to be once pain is manageable, if you try to get back too soon then you start the cycle of irritation and inflammation again. Think of it as an angry wasp, it doesn't take much to make it angry but takes quite a while for it to calm down. Once you have been walking pain-free, stairs don't hurt and you have tried the odd jog, all without pain, then follow the rehab run principle: 3 minutes of moderate paced running, followed by 2 minutes of stretches to the abductors and glutes. Repeat 5 times if pain-free, stop if pain returns at any stage.

Groin or adductor strain

What is it?

First of all, the groin is not a muscle, nor is there a single muscle in the body with the term 'groin' in it. So where does the term groin strain come from? Groin is a term that identifies the inguinal canal, which is the area between the abdomen and the thigh. When physios talk of the groin, we are talking about the origins of the adductor muscles, which are those that sit on the inside of the thigh and pull the leg inwards, like bringing your leg into the car. The muscles are called adductor longus, adductor brevis and adductor magnus, gracilis and pectineus.

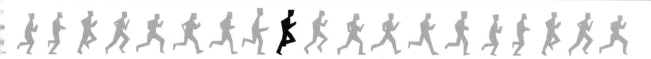

COMMON REASONS FOR INJURY

Runners tend not to get this injury when running, but instead usually get it from participating in other sports. Whilst the adductors are used during running, they are often quite weak compared to the prime movers in the running technique. When a runner then takes to playing sports such as football or rugby, the groin is a weak spot and prone to injury. Then every movement including that of running will be too painful to perform.

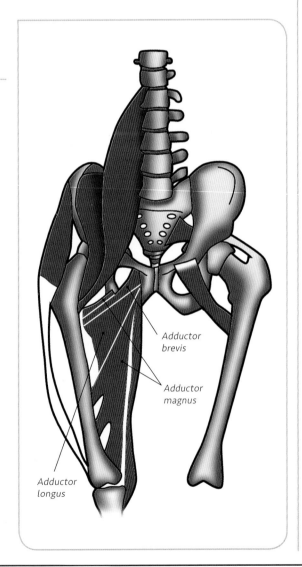

Adductor brevis

Adductor magnus

Adductor longus

EARLY WARNING SIGNS

- A sharp pull in the groin area followed by immediate pain
- Pain squeezing legs together
- Pain moving leg inwards towards the midline
- Pain turning in bed.

PROGRESSION OF INJURY

The pain doesn't really get worse unless you injure it again, but, like the bursa (see page 145), it has a high irritability, which means that with very little stimuli the pain is back. Even just taking a flight of stairs too fast can cause the pain to rush back and more injury to occur. You have to be very careful to protect this area and keep it safe from further injury.

SELF-ASSESSMENT

Sit with the sides of your feet touching and gradually and slowly allow your knees to drop out to the sides. If you feel pain in the injured side, it is likely you have hurt your groin.

Secondly, you can stand side on a step and abduct your leg so that the medial edge of your foot rests along the length of the step. Now lean in towards the step and compare to the other side. Pain in the groin area suggests an injury to the adductor muscle's origin, commonly referred to as the groin.

TREATMENT

Massage to the adductor muscles and deep transverse frictions to the site of injury, for two minutes until the area feels less pain and then up to 10 minutes for the therapy to the tendon. Between treatments you will be expected to perform gentle stretching and some basic strengthening exercises as outlined below.

SELF-TREATMENT

Choose exercises: Hip flexors (stretch), page 173, Hamstring (stretch), page 178, ITB Tensor fascia latae (stretch), page 178, Swiss ball abduction in side plank, page 180, and Quads foam rolling, page 181.

It's important to do the resisted hip abduction in an eccentric muscle contraction, slowly returning to neutral at each repetition.

WHAT TO EXPECT FROM A PHYSIOTHERAPIST

The treatment is similar to that of other muscle and tendon injuries, using deep transverse frictions and massage to good effect. This is in a particularly personal area, so be prepared to pull your own towel high up under your shorts to reveal as much as possible of the inner thigh for the physio to

PRACTITIONER PROTOCOL

- Soft tissue massage to the adductors combined with eccentric loading of the adductors are a great combination, but the patient has to avoid aggravating activities
- DTF to the origin are of great use, but not all patients are going to feel comfortable with this treatment
- Recently, shockwave therapy to the area has proven excellent (anecdotally) for this injury with return to playing football within 4 weeks. 500 shocks at 10 per second using 1.5Htz, followed by 2000 shocks at 10 per second using 2.5Htz. 4 sessions 1 week apart.

CLIENT STORY: LEE, 32

I have always played sport to a high level, playing football for Carlisle schoolboys and also for my county. I ran the 100m and 200m at county-level and held the 200m junior track record at county level for many years, and have also enjoyed long-distance running too.

During my sporting life I have fortunately been relatively injury-free, though I have had Achilles tendonitis and the odd pulled muscle, which I have always found very frustrating. I booked in to see Paul after pulling my groin in a pre-season football match. My groin was very painful when walking and excruciating when trying to kick the ball. I feared that I would miss a large part of the season with the injury, not to mention my enjoyment of running, and a few winter races I had planned.

During my first visit to see Paul my groin was extremely painful when touched and so we decided to treat it with shockwave therapy based upon the benefits of tissue healing and pain relief. This is a therapy I had not heard of before but

I was interested to see the effects and trusted Paul's opinion. The next day I could not believe the difference. There was still considerable pain, but it felt so much better than before, it felt like a miracle.

Stupidly, I tried to play football that weekend, however, this only lasted 25min before the pain was back, although I have to say it wasn't as bad this time. I then decided to be more sensible and commit to the treatment. I had four sessions of shockwave therapy in total and after the third session I tried a run, which to my amazement was pain-free. Later that week I managed to play football for a full 90mins, running and turning as hard as I liked, to both mine and my team mates' amazement.

I was fully back running and football training and remaining pain free in a fraction of the time I have seen in any other groin strain sufferer I am amazed how well the treatment worked and my fellow sporting colleagues are also astonished by the results.

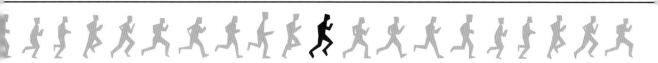

work on. The groin origins are on the lower bones of the pelvis and as such some of the closest muscles to the reproductive organs, so please discuss any concerns you may have with your physiotherapist before treatment begins. Physios are used to this sort of treatment and whilst we work hard to make sure you are comfortable, it can be a new experience for you and we are ever mindful of this.

GETTING BACK TO RUNNING

This requires time and steady running, but in fact, unlike the bursa issue, it is possible to run a lot earlier than you might expect. The issue is you can't really run on uneven ground and you will most likely be running with a slightly shorter stride whilst the healing takes place. Regular stretches will ensure that you do not lose range for when you have fully rehabilitated the area.

High hamstring tendinopathy

What is it?

A few years ago I barely had a hamstring to deal with on a day-to-day basis, but these days I have runners of all abilities coming in with 'high hamstring tendinopathies'.

What does this mean? Well, the hamstrings originate from your seat bones (Ischial tuberosities) and travel down the leg to the knee joint, attaching just beyond to the uppermost tibia and fibula of the lower leg.

There are three hamstrings: the biceps femoris on the lateral side (attaching to the fibula), and the semitendinosus and semimembranosus, both of which attach medially to the tibia.

The hamstrings have some weak spots: the attachment at the ischial tuberosities (the seat bones), the point at which the tendon becomes muscle (the myotendon junction); the central belly muscle, and then the attachment at the knee joint.

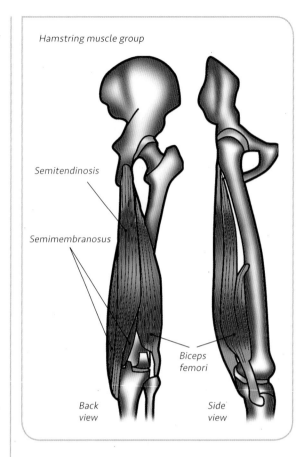

Hamstring muscle group

Semitendinosis

Semimembranosus

Biceps femori

Back view   *Side view*

The origin at the ischial tuberosities also comes with a small bursa (a fluid-filled sac) to reduce friction between the tendon and the bone on movement. These can become irritated with chronically tight hamstrings and cause a great deal of pain. The hamstrings are supplied by the sciatic nerve, so any compression of the nerve radiates pain along the muscle itself. The tendon can injure causing a tendinopathy (previously known as tendinosis – see page 89 for more info on name change) which is pain with every step you take, often worsening over time.

Think of tendons as your most boring friend, afraid and resistant to change. A step up in your training programme, an increase in strength training, or a movement to the track or hill reps is enough for a hamstring tendon to become unhappy.

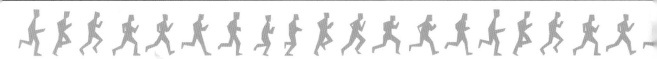

EARLY WARNING SIGNS

- Pain high up at the top of the hamstring
- Pain in the buttock on the same side
- Restricted movement into trunk flexion
- Pain on hamstring stretches
- Pain on hamstring activity.

COMMON REASONS FOR INJURY

I see the majority of these injuries in the first quarter of the year, as athletes come from the road and trails back onto the track and start to run in a circular motion, always in the same direction, for hours on end. Usually, track sessions also mean a change in footwear, to a more minimalist, less supportive shoe. All these factors seem to increase the number of treatments for right-side high hamstring tendinopathies, stressed by the repetitive nature of running track bends in the same direction time and time again.

PROGRESSION OF INJURY

The hamstring pain will be quite mild at first and not like a sudden pull. As it is usually a chronic injury the progression can be quite slow. Many people present with this as glute pain rather than identifying it as hamstring pain. The pain gets worse and worse until you feel like you cannot sit down. Usually however, with a good warm-up most people feel they can continue to run. The pain can feel like it is very deep and close to the more personal areas of the body, sometimes people decide not to go for treatment for a long time because of this. Early intervention is always best and treatments are very good these days.

SELF-ASSESSMENT

Try a hamstring (stretch), page 178, and compare each side to see if the pain is high up on the injured side, not to be confused with a tight muscle; the pain will be very specifically under the glute muscle, many confuse this with a glute muscle injury.

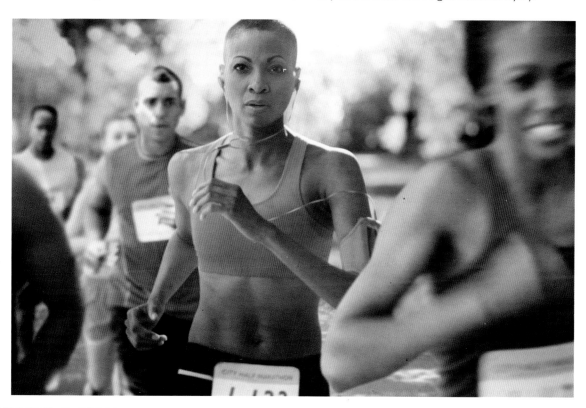

Piriformis syndrome

What is it?

Piriformis syndrome is an injury that presents in almost all cases by someone coming into the clinic announcing that they have sciatica. Sciatica is a low back injury that causes referred pain along the back of the legs and is quite debilitating. Piriformis syndrome is when the piriformis muscle becomes tight and because it overlies the sciatic nerve within the pelvis, it causes pressure on the nerve and can therefore provide some of the same symptoms – referred pain along the back of the legs, pain in the buttocks and even pain in the lateral lower leg or ankle.

The piriformis runs from the sacrum, the inverted triangular-shaped area at the base of the spine, to the top of the femur (thigh bone). It externally rotates the leg during hip extension and abducts the hip during flexion. It has a weird additional element in that it will adduct the hip if the knee is flexed beyond 90 degrees. In the main, think of it as a hip external rotator – if a piriformis is very tight then the person will feel happier with the foot turned out slightly to offload the muscle.

With piriformis syndrome the patient will often say their referral symptoms down the leg are worse when sitting and driving the car. This makes sense, as there is compression of the muscle but also the hip is often flexed beyond 90 degrees in a car seat, and yet the knee generally falls outwards from the midline into abduction, causing more tension on

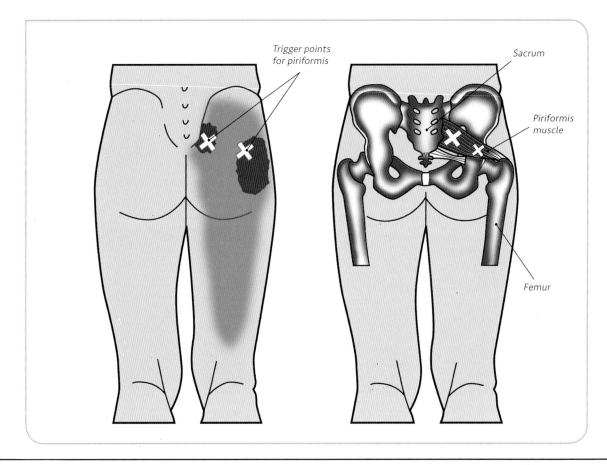

Trigger points for piriformis

Sacrum

Piriformis muscle

Femur

the piriformis as the muscle acts as an adductor in this position.

EARLY WARNING SIGNS

- Pain in the glute
- Pain along the back of the leg
- Pain travelling down the leg when seated
- Pain becoming worse when running
- Symptoms seem to match those of sciatica.

COMMON REASONS FOR THE INJURY

Piriformis syndrome is common for those who do not have an effective stretch routine, who spend a long time seated for work or long periods sat in a car. There is a small percentage of people whose sciatic nerves actually pass through their piriformis muscle and therefore much less tension would be needed in this muscle to impinge on the nerve.

Lots of running, especially where you have the wrong footwear, or poor biomechanics, can cause the piriformis muscle to be overworked; it then tightens and impinges on the sciatic nerve causing pain.

PROGRESSION OF THE INJURY

The symptoms become more and more severe and sufferers find it difficult to take even the shortest of car journeys, often having to take breaks and getting out after just a few minutes. Sitting at a desk becomes very difficult and they start to fidget all the time. The sciatic-type pain continues to worsen and eventually becomes unremitting and plays out just like a bulging disk.

SELF-ASSESSMENT

Pull your leg towards you to stretch the piriformis: Piriformis stretch, page 183. If you get more pain with the injured side then hold the stretch for 3 x 45 seconds. Afterwards perform Sciatic nerve flossing, page 180, and then perform the stretch again. Compare the feeling you have before and after the flossing.

An improvement in your symptoms will suggest there is some compromise of the sciatic nerve at the piriformis muscle level. You may find that repetitions

of the above reduce your symptoms significantly, but this has not addressed any underlying biomechanical issues you might have.

TREATMENT

Treatment for piriformis syndrome is deep tissue work and stretches to the muscle, and using trigger point techniques to reduce in size the muscle knots that serve to make the muscle shorter. Acupuncture can be a useful tool to try to get deep into the muscle and reduce the size of those trigger points. Once pain has been reduced and there is less referral pain, you can start to nerve floss, which is a rather underwhelming exercise whereby you slide the sciatic nerve through the soft tissues to ensure its function is optimized (page 180). Daily stretching is required for the piriformis, with treatments usually at weekly intervals.

SELF-TREATMENT

Stretching the piriformis can be done in many ways. To get the best stretch you need the knee to be pulled up high towards your chest with your lower leg being rotated around at the same time. All of these positions really work and can be fitted into your daily routine. The essence of a good stretch programme for the piriformis is to try a variety of different positions and stretches to ensure you stretch it through its various ranges.

Choose the following stretches: The clam – hip abduction/rotation (strength), page 173, Glute activation (strength), page 175, Core muscles (strength), page 176, Glutes (stretch), page 177, Hamstring (stretch), page 178 and of course Piriformis stretch, page 183.

WHAT TO EXPECT FROM A PHYSIOTHERAPIST

The piriformis is a deep muscle in the glutes, so expect to have some pretty intensive work performed on your backside. It's totally your choice but I genuinely feel that there is a much better treatment available if you are prepared to expose a bit of glute for a physio to work on. I completely understand that not everyone is an exhibitionist

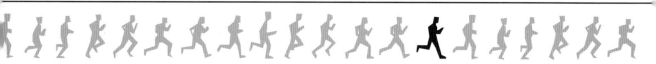

Can deep massage and stretching truly reach the deep piriformis muscle successfully? If you try these treatments alone, then you may enjoy limited success. You may wish to try some medical acupuncture/dry needling deep into the tissues as well.

The real benefit to this injury comes from daily mobilizing of the sciatic nerve when combined with the stretches to piriformis. However, these positive changes will be transient in the absence of correcting the biomechanical fault that underlies the cause. Check for pelvic alignment, leg length and a full assessment of the range of movement and strength from the lower back all the way to the foot and ankle mechanics.

It may well take a long time to work through the long list of issues that present but systematically address these one by one, applying treatments according to the findings of your assessments. Check especially for glute max firing and core strength.

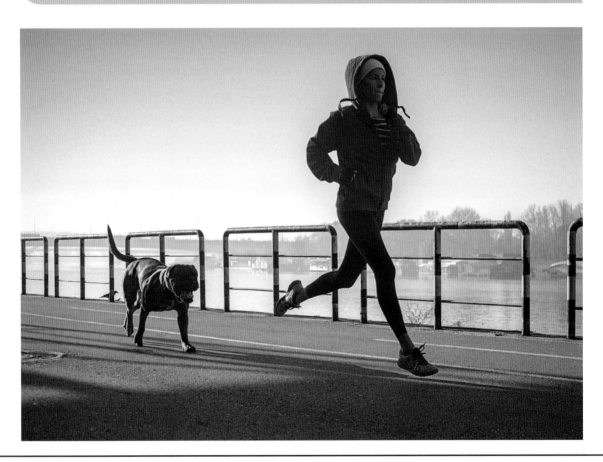

I have been running for nearly 30 years, initially for weight loss and then a little more seriously as my career began in the fitness industry. I became a personal fitness trainer in 1996, having been a keen gym bunny for a few years, but I never stopped running, although I didn't bother with races much until around 2004, when I decided to give triathlons a go.

My first marathon was as part of Ironman Nice in 2007 and I didn't go back to that distance until I entered the first running of the Kielder marathon in Northumberland in October 2010; completing it in 3 hours 58mins. I went back to the same race the following year with a niggling injury that I didn't deal with, which I subsequently have realized was the start of my piriformis issues, and finished in 4hrs 6mins. Rather than deal with my injuries properly I decided to go long in 2012 and signed up for the North Downs Way 50-mile run in August of that year, entering a 30-mile run in the New Forest in May and a 40-miler in June as part of my training. Feeling like I had a score to settle with Kielder I also entered that to round my year off.

In an attempt to get the miles in I ignored any other form of training and just ran, aiming for time on my feet rather than pace, but in June the wheels fell off. On the 40-mile run I made it to about 26 miles before I had to stop in agony, convinced I had a stress fracture in my left shin. Unsure of what to do I rested for a while but on a visit to my family home my sister told me about a new physio in the area.

It only took Paul a few minutes to diagnose me with piriformis syndrome and to set about treating me. Thankfully he didn't tell me I couldn't run but sent me home with some serious stretching and rehab work to do and I continued to see him, initially on a weekly basis up to the 50-mile run in August.

Having been almost convinced I wouldn't be able to run I got to the start line and completed the event, stopping at all the aid stations along the route to do my stretches, in just under 12 hours. Even though I was not injury-free I decided to do Kielder that year and finished in a slower time of 4hrs 16mins. However, I took the rest of the year off, carried on my treatments with Paul until I was running pain-free, changed my running programme so that I was running smarter not harder and came back to Kielder stronger in 2013. Because I was injury-free throughout my training, thanks to Paul's advice and treatments, I was able to train harder and more consistently. On the same course I knocked 29mins off my course record; completing it in 3hrs 29mins, coming first in my age group (40–44) and the fifth woman overall.

157

triathlete, so feel free to wear some thin shorts for the physio to work through and we will do our best. The treatment requires some trigger point work as well as deep transverse frictions. Trigger points are hyper-irritable sections of fascia surrounding the skeletal muscle. Pressure placed directly on the trigger point, known as ischemic compression, produces pain. The theory behind ischemic compression is that without a blood supply and all the nutrients that this provides the trigger point cannot remain active. Subsequent stretching to elongate the fibres produces the therapeutic element of the treatment and home stretching prolongs the effects between treatments.

GETTING BACK TO RUNNING

In some cases it can be instant. The pain relief felt is measurable in clinic and yet if the cause of the injury in the first place is a fault in the biomechanics or the footwear used, then unless these issues are addressed you will faced by an ongoing cycle of treatment, running, pain, treatment. In this event, make sure you have a full gait analysis to assess your footwear and biomechanics.

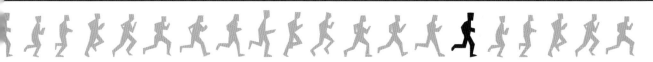

Iliopsoas bursitis

What is it?

Anterior hip pain for a runner generally comes in the form of bursitis of the iliopsoas bursa. The bursa is a fluid filled sac, the job of which is to reduce friction between the tendon and any neighbouring bone. (I refer to them as puffer fish, calm and functional when undisturbed but violent, swollen and angry when irritated.) The bursae tend to stay inflamed and painful for some time after the biomechanical assault has ended, causing long-lasting pain and aggravation on movement. Hip flexors are a group of

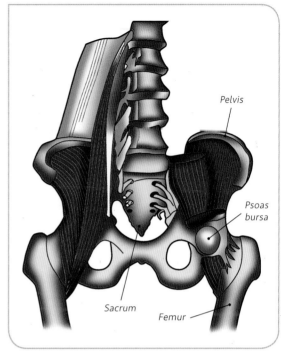

muscles, namely the tensor fascia latae (TFL) which is the contractile portion of the iliotibial band (ITB) iliacus, psoas major and rectus femoris, one of the quads that also acts as a hip flexor.

Let's talk at first about psoas major and iliacus, known together as iliopsoas. The iliopsoas is a hip flexor that originates (psoas major) from the lower thoracic and all of the lumbar vertebral bodies and disks and attaches to the top of the femur. It provides movements of hip flexion, but when the femur is fixed, also flexion of the spine. It is a very strong muscle that can be the cause of low back pain when it becomes too tight. Served by the same nerve supply as the male testicles there have been occasions where tight psoas muscles have referred pain to this area setting off some worrying thoughts.

EARLY WARNING SIGNS

- Anterior hip pain, especially when running or straight afterwards
- Referral pain into the anterior thigh, quads muscle, or into the glutes

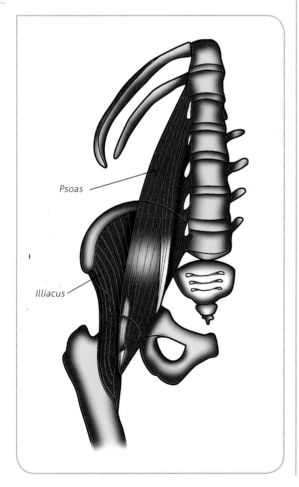

- Tenderness into the quads muscles and anterior hip area when touched
- For the male, possible referral pain to the testes.

COMMON REASONS FOR INJURY

The hip flexor is one of the main muscle protagonists in many injuries. The hip flexor doesn't work alone when flexing the hip, it is helped by the main quadriceps muscle, the rectus femoris, which crosses both the hip and knee joint, thus having more than one function. Hip flexor soreness is fairly common owing to the changes that occur in the muscle between sitting at a desk and going for a run. The flexed hip position when sitting is causing a shortening of the muscle, but the posture work the muscle must elicit to keep you from slouching is huge and so it is being worked all day long (unless you slouch in your work chair).

Therefore when we move from hours sat at a desk with little respite or stretching and ask this poor little muscle to go for a run we are expecting a lot. You need 90 degrees of hip extension to stand up from a seated position and then another 15 or so degrees of hip extension during your running gait. It's quite easy to see how runners end up with problems with their iliopsoas bursa and low back pain given the differing roles of the muscle group in this daily routine.

PROGRESSION OF THE INJURY

Consider the attachments once again. The psoas major comes from the lower back. The lower back is curved convex into the lumbar lordosis. As you extend your leg on a tight psoas from all day sat at your desk, you pull on that lumbar portion of the back. The psoas being a strong muscle, it is more resilient than your lumbar spine or the supporting muscles and therefore can cause pain from a multitude of irregular movement patterns and stress.

Add to this what we know about the effect of a flexed hip on the position of the knee. A tight hip flexor component will make it hard to fully extend the hip and thus overload the knee, potentially causing PFPS. You may never notice the back tension,

or write it off as spending long periods at your desk and in your car, however, the potentially debilitating knee pain will have you foam rolling your ITB and taping everything from your groin to your shin, when what you really need is more breaks from your desk and a hip flexor stretch or two during the day.

SELF-ASSESSMENT

Pull your bent knee up towards your chest and at the same time bring it across the body to compress the anterior hip. Pain deep within the hip is a sign of an inflamed bursa in the front of the hip.

TREATMENT

Treatment of the hip flexor is not just about restoring length and therefore a more functional range of movement, you also need to be sure that you are not overloading the lumbar spine, and correct any postural changes during sitting, standing, walking and of course running. Usually there is treatment also to the quadriceps muscle and checks to ensure that the glutes are strong and firing correctly. The physiotherapy treatment for a psoas muscle issue is as much about the biomechanics of the individual as it is the local muscular problems that present. To make this difficult task as simple as possible the following self-treatment exercises will ensure that you tackle the most obvious areas that require improvement, meaning that you will have a greater than 50% chance of being able to fix this issue yourself (provided you do not have a complex issue).

SELF-TREATMENT

Choose the following exercises: Hip flexors (stretch), page 173, Hip adductors (stretch), page 174, Glute activation (strength), page 175, Core muscles (strength), page 176, Quads foam rolling, page 181 and Quads stretch, page 182.

WHAT TO EXPECT FROM A PHYSIOTHERAPIST

When you visit a physiotherapist, the initial questions and tests will be looking for pain in the anterior hip during contraction of the hip flexors

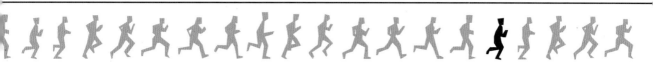

PRACTITIONER PROTOCOL

An injection can be very useful for the quick reduction of symptoms here, however, what is the underlying cause of the pain? A full biomechanics review is needed. The pain usually comes on gradually over time and assessment is muddled with some passive and some active tests eliciting pain, but not all. Use the information you have from these tests alongside your hip and pelvis assessment to make an informed judgment as to the cause.

If in doubt, strengthen what is weak and lengthen what is loose, but always check the pelvic alignment and the tension/tenderness in the inguinal ligament.

Useful exercises are Single leg balance, page 171, The clam – hip abduction/rotation (strength), page 173, Hip flexors (stretch), page 173, Hip adductors (stretch), page 174, Hamstrings (strength), page 174, Glute activation (strength), page 175, Core muscles (strength), page 176, Glutes (stretch), page 177 and Quads stretch, page 182.

and/or quads muscles and tenderness when the psoas is palpated.

Once diagnosed the physiotherapist needs to decide if this is a biomechanical issue or if the psoas has flared up through training or just a tight muscle. Testing will not only be localized to the hip, the whole functional foot, ankle, hip and lower back will need to be assessed.

You may benefit from orthotic devices, but in the main gentle stretching of the hip flexors and strengthening of the glutes and core will be prescribed.

For persistent injuries of this nature, a steroid injection into the bursa can reduce it in size and enable more commitment to the exercises mentioned as you work towards a full recovery.

GETTING BACK TO RUNNING

The reason you will have suffered this injury in the first place is the repetitive movement of running. You must be confident that the bursa has settled down before commencing a new running programme. I suggest starting very slowly and building up from 5 sets of 3 minutes at first, that way you can stop and stretch your psoas (Hip flexors (stretch), page ***) each rest stop. If that goes OK, then rest for

a day or two then repeat but this time 5 sets of 4 minutes. You can continue to build on this provided you are pain free and recover well. Continue with the rehabilitation exercises for at least a few weeks once you are back into your training.

Low back pain

Low back pain is one of the most common ailments across the globe, not just for runners but for all members of the population. As much as 80% of the population can expect a bout of low back pain within their lifetime (Macfarlane *et al.*, 1999). For runners it may well be less, but definitive research isn't available.

I think that low back pain is a fitting subject to finish off a book on running injuries as it really bridges the gap between running-specific injury and injury sustained by the general population.

What is it?

Low back pain is felt in the lower ⅓ of the spine. It can be central, or to one side. Symptoms can range from a sharp, very localized pain through to a

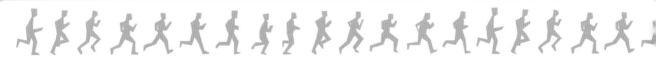

diffuse, widespread ache. Both pains can come with or without referred pain. Referred pain is pain that is felt elsewhere other than the site of the injury. It is quite complicated to explain referred pain to patients – there may not in fact be any pain at the main site of injury – and so it's a huge leap of faith for someone to take when visiting a physiotherapist to have their glute worked on for a pain that feels totally isolated in the ankle.

Mainly, however, with low back pain in runners, if there is some referred pain as well as in the back, then it is most commonly found into the glute and

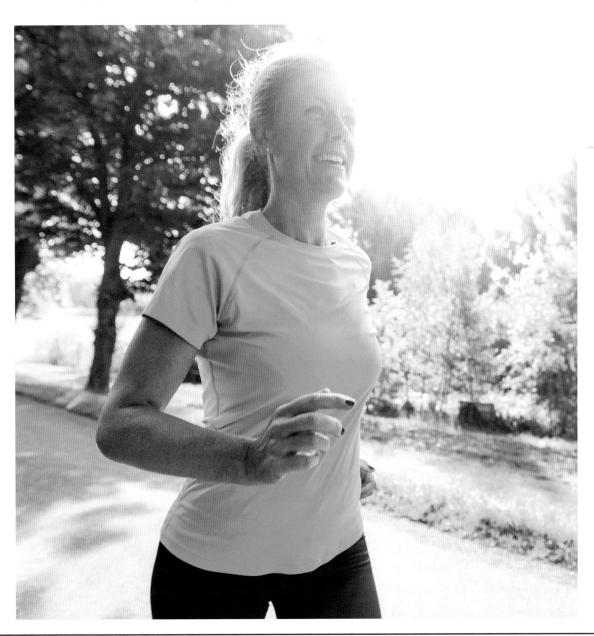

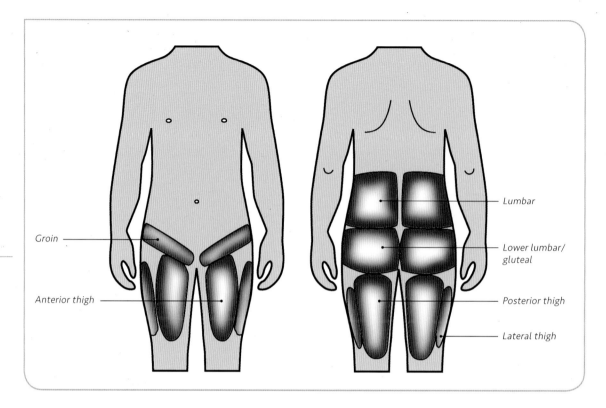

Groin

Anterior thigh

Lumbar

Lower lumbar/ gluteal

Posterior thigh

Lateral thigh

upper hamstring area. However, pain can also be felt into the anterior thigh, down the side of the leg and into the groin area.

EARLY WARNING SIGNS

- Pain felt specifically in the lower back
- Pain felt in the lower back when moving the hip/ leg
- Pain felt in the lower back and also in the glutes and legs
- Pins and needles in the glutes or legs
- Numbness in the glutes and legs.

There are some 'red flags' to look out for with your back pain, which mean you need to take some immediate action:

- Numbness in your saddle area (the area between your legs that would make contact with a horse saddle when riding)

- Loss of bladder or bowel control or urinary retention
- Significant loss of strength in your legs.

You should seek emergency medical care if you experience these red flag symptoms, especially if you have a first bout of back pain and are under 16 years of age or over 50 years of age. These symptoms could suggest an impingement of the spinal cord which is a medical emergency. If these symptoms are clearly there, then please get yourself looked at immediately.

If, however, you are confident that you have a fairly standard low back pain and have visited your GP to confirm there is no underlying cause, the following information will be useful to you.

COMMON REASONS FOR THE INJURY

With runners the first things a physio will want to do for central low back pain are to assess the posture,

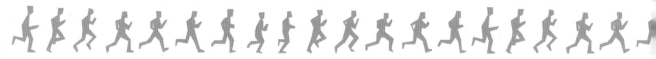

and then the length of neighbouring muscles (particularly hamstrings, glutes and hip flexors). This is because runners are terrible at stretching. Look around at your club mates and see how many actually spend any real time stretching between training sessions or at the end of the training session. It is my experience in clinic that only 25% of runners will have a good attitude to muscle length and injury prevention, the rest just want to use all the available time they have out running, so something has to give.

The hamstrings originate from the ischial tuberosities, or seat bones. When tight they provide a force to pull the pelvis into posterior tilt, pulling the pelvis lower at the back and flattening the lumbar curvature. This resultant stress on the low back can cause pain.

The glutes, particularly piriformis, can pull tight across the neighbouring sciatic nerve and cause referred pain along the back of the leg.

The psoas hip flexor muscles, as previously described (see page 158), originate from the lumbar spine (the lower portion) and then attach to the top of the thigh bone, so when the muscle activates it flexes the hip. If this muscle becomes tight, then it can pull on the lumbar spine and bring about low back pain. So to start by testing these three structures for length, then reducing tension where necessary, may well alleviate the low back pain. Consider the movement when running as the hip is pulled into extension (right).

The tight hip flexor will pull on the lower portion of the spine at its origin. These simple mechanical changes have a huge impact on your injury potential at the lower back. Conversely during hip flexion, the hamstrings are being pulled tight and the resultant force on the pelvis can cause pain.

Low back pain has many causes and contributing factors such as tight hip flexors and tight hamstrings. Glutes also need looking at as part of the diagnosis. It may be worth while taking a look at the chapters in this book that cover hamstrings, hip flexors and glutes for an alternative diagnosis to your low back pain. It is the role of the physiotherapist to work through his or her testing of each to decide whether the problem is coming from the low back or locally at the muscle or tendon.

PROGRESSION OF THE INJURY

Low back pain tends to get worse rather than better. In the really chronic cases where there was no actual incident when the pain started, the pain will wax and wane throughout the days, weeks and years, making it possible for you to function at an almost normal level for 80% of the time. Cases that are acute need more medical attention and are not covered here.

The variations of low back pain are so many that, for the rest of this section, the advice is there to try to help those specifically with an ongoing, nagging low back pain.

SELF-ASSESSMENT

The symptoms of low back pain are so varied that we have to stay specific to common running-based complaints.

See if your pain is reduced when you bring your knees closer to your chest. Does your pain worsen when you straighten your legs? If you perform Hip flexors (stretch), page 173, do you feel significant pain in the anterior hip? If the answers to the above are both a resounding yes, then your back pain may well be due to tight hip flexors.

However, if you are getting low back pain that is worse when you lean back and especially when you combine this extension with some rotation and side bend, then you will be loading the facet joints within the spine. Performing the same test to the opposite side may well be pain free, suggesting that one of the spinal joints has some inflammation around the smaller articulation of the spinal segment.

Of course if your low back pain is more than a niggle, don't even try to self-diagnose. Take yourself off to see a physiotherapist and let them do some testing.

TREATMENT

The treatment protocol has so many variations because there are so many possible causes of low back pain. Typically it will include some soft tissue massage, spinal mobilizations

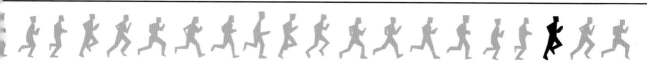

(fairly gentle pressing on the spinal segments) and if required and you agree to them, some spinal manipulations, during which a slight clicking sound is heard. Contrary to popular belief, this isn't a segment of your back moving from one place to another; you weren't 'out of place' beforehand. It's much more likely to be a slight change in pressure within the joint that has a therapeutic effect and can develop movement at that level, previously reduced owing to muscle spasm or joint pressure. Spinal mobilizations and spinal manipulation are shown to the right.

You will have a few exercises to get on with at home. Little and often works best with back pain, so be prepared to adjust your diary to make time regularly throughout the day if you want to get better.

SELF-TREATMENT
Perform the following exercises: Hip flexors (stretch), page 173, Glute activation (strength), page 175, Core muscles (strength), page 176,

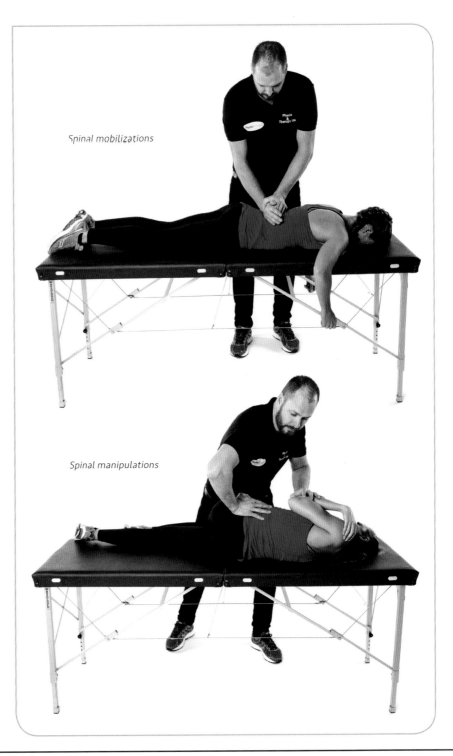

Spinal mobilizations

Spinal manipulations

PRACTITIONER PROTOCOL

The treatment protocols are so varied because of the sheer number of reasons and pathologies for low back pain. However, make sure that when working with runners you consider the following:

- Core strength
- Hip flexor length
- Glute strength and timing
- Pelvic stability
- Gait analysis

- Footwear choice and age/usage
- Hamstring tension/strength
- Posture, particularly the upper body
- Gastroc and soleus length and foot mechanics including hallux rigidus.

Glutes (stretch), page 177, Hamstring (stretch), page 178, Sciatic nerve flossing, page 180 and McKenzie back extensions, page 184.

WHAT TO EXPECT FROM A PHYSIOTHERAPIST

When you visit the physiotherapist, you will be examined for posture, alignment and flexibility. The best clothing is some shorts and a vest top so we can see as many of the moving parts as possible. It is absolutely necessary to lift the top up and ideally for men we would remove the top altogether. You need to wear what is comfortable for you, but the more the physio can see of your back the better.

Within your pain limits it is good to see how far you can bend and flex the trunk, with clear signals to when you feel the pain come on and to what level (0–10). From this information we can work out where the pain is coming from and therefore direct the treatment to the source of the injury (not always where you are feeling the pain). Then we can retest and hopefully show some reduction in pain from start to finish.

GETTING BACK TO RUNNING

Returning to running is a simple equation of pain versus movement. If it hurts to walk, then you usually cannot consider running very far. There is a great deal of scientific evidence to support exercise in any form as a great way to manage low back pain, but if you are experiencing too much pain to function, your desire or ability to run is pretty much gone for a while. If you are considering a run, clearly you have less pain now and so you would want to ease into this gently. Assuming that you have spent some time on the exercises prescribed by your physiotherapist and they are happy for you to return gently, then try 10 minutes at first, then wait to see if there is a reaction afterwards for a day or so, then try 15 or 20 minutes and so on. You need to test the water gently as often the pain will come on as a reaction to the run, not during the run itself.

THE HIP AND PELVIS

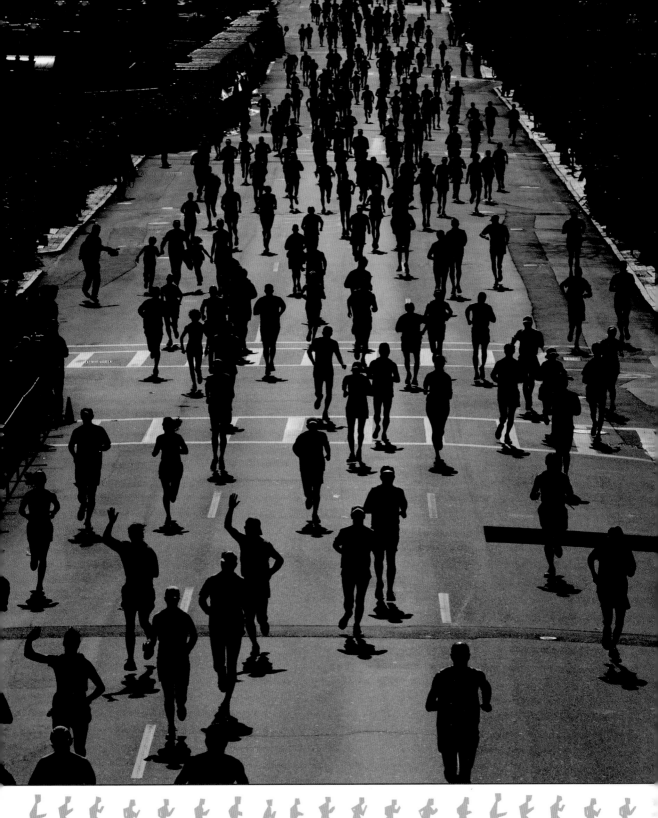

APPENDIX 1

REHABILITATION EXERCISES

Towel grabbing
(STRENGTH) TIME: 2 MINUTES

This exercise helps to build the strength through the arch of the foot as well as having a neuromuscular benefit by exciting the nerves for improved all-round function.

- Place a towel out on the floor in front of your chair
- Place the toes onto the towel with the heel flat on the floor
- By raising and lowering your forefoot, grab the towel with your toes on every downward movement and scrunch the towel towards you
- Repeat this for two minutes.

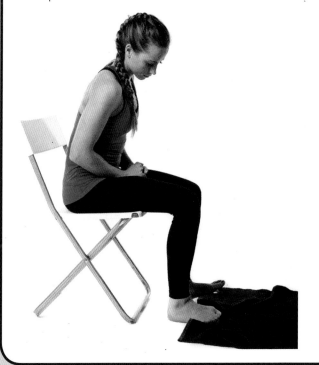
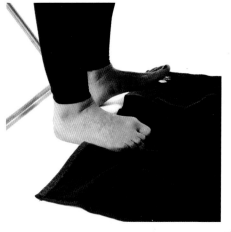

Calf

(STRETCH) TIME: 1.5 MINUTES

A static stretch as part of your prehab is still very relevant, although dynamic stretching as part of a warm-up is now favoured. Static stretching is where you place the muscle under tension and hold that position for a time, dynamic stretching is increasing the range of movement through a series of repeated movements.

- Hold the stretch for 45 seconds x 3 per day
- Place the foot of the injured side against the wall so the toes are just above the height of a skirting board/baseboard
- The heel should be a few centimetres away from the wall (the foot at approximately a 45-degree angle)
- Then use the back foot to push you gently forwards, thus bringing your knee towards the wall.

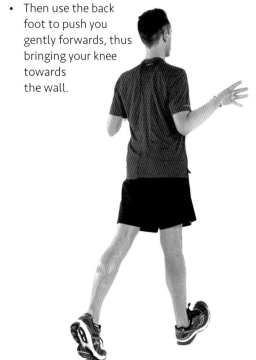

Soleus

(STRETCH) TIME: 1.5 MINUTES

Stretch your soleus (the deeper flat muscle in the calf) for 45 seconds each leg. Stand facing a wall with your feet 10–20cms from the wall, one foot in front of the other. Bend both knees until you feel a dull stretch deep in the calf muscle.

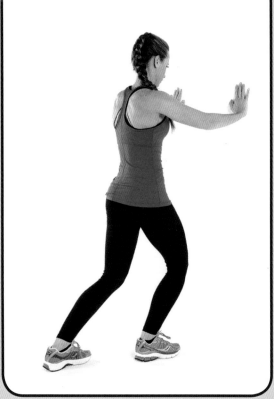

Calf raises

(STRENGTH) TIME: 3 MINUTES

- Start on your tiptoes standing on the edge of a step
- Slowly lower down until your heel cannot lower any further
- Return to the top again in one smooth movement
- Repeat 3 x 15 reps.

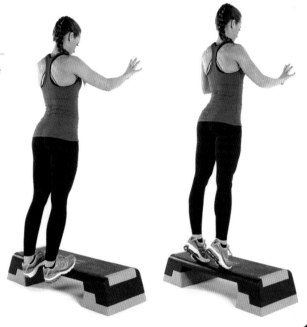

Toe raises

(STRENGTH) TIME: 3 MINUTES

- Stand with your back against a wall
- Take a step away from the wall
- Keeping your heels in contact with the floor, raise your toes up as far as you can and slowly lower back towards the floor, but do not allow them to touch
- Repeat 4 x 25 reps.

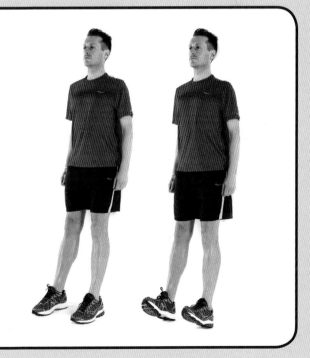

Tibialis posterior
(STRENGTH) TIME: 3 MINUTES

This is a strength exercise for those wanting to reduce over-pronation and the risk of shin splints.

- Start with the toes pointing outward, then raise the heels up
- When close to the top of your calf raise, rotate the heels in toward each other before slowly lowering them back down to flat again
- Repeat these 25 reps x 3.

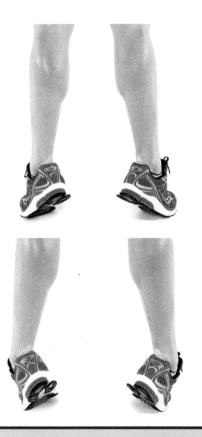

Peroneals–ankle eversion
(STRENGTH) TIME: 4 MINUTES

- Tie a loop into a stretchy exercise band
- Place the loop over the foot to be worked
- Hook the remaining length of band around the other foot and pull the free end towards you
- Twist the long lateral edge of your foot out to the side against the resistance
- Don't rotate around the ankle. The big toe should remain roughly in line with the shinbone with little or no rotation of the foot laterally
- Push out against the resistance of the band 15 times x 3, returning to the resting position at the end of each repetition.

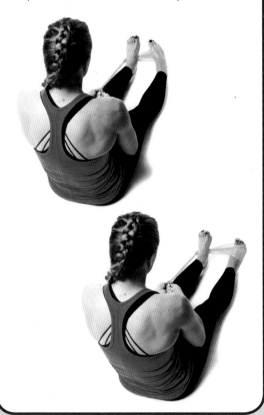

Shin

(STRETCH) TIME: 1 MINUTE

Place your knee on top of a foam roller with your toes pointed back. Gradually increase the stretch by lowering your hips to the floor. Hold the stretch for 30–40 seconds.

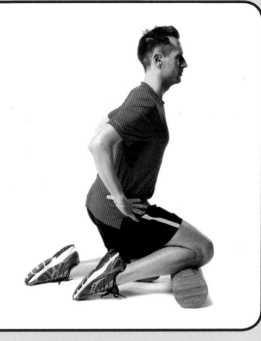

Single leg balance

TIME: 2–4 MINUTES

- Balance on a cushion or pillow on one leg
- Hold the free leg in a variety of positions used through the running action
- Use arms to alter your centre of gravity by moving them slowly into alternating positions as if running
- Work hard to maintain the balance through the foot, ankle, knee and hip
- Keep your hips level throughout
- Balance for 20–60 seconds and repeat with the other leg.

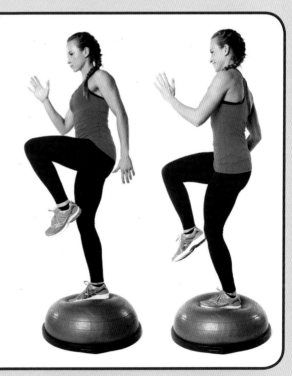

Variation on the single leg balance: BOSU® lunge
TIME: 4 MINUTES

The BOSU® lunge is an extension of the prior exercise and can be used instead of the basic move once you have attained a suitable level of balance.

- Place a BOSU® plastic side down and stand a generous stride away from the centre of the apparatus
- Step forwards placing one foot onto the centre of the pod
- Bend both knees and then push back to standing
- Alternate the lead leg for 15 reps each.

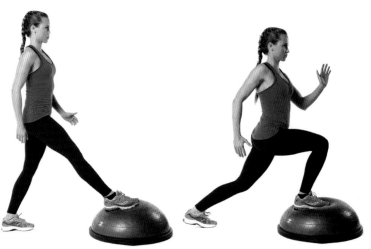

Variation on the single leg balance: lunge into single leg balance
TIME: 4 MINUTES

Combine the single leg balance with the BOSU® lunge for a functional exercise that works the full running action and encompasses strength to the core, upper back, shoulders, neck, as well as the foot, ankle, knee, hip and glutes.

- Lunge onto the BOSU®
- Lower hands (holding a weight if desired)
- At the same time lift the trail leg off the floor
- Balance for 3 seconds and return to the start position
- Repeat alternating legs for 15 reps each side
- Lift up onto your tiptoes
- Slowly lower down.

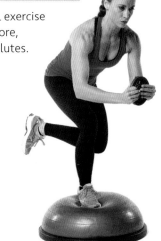

The clam – hip abduction/rotation

(STRENGTH) TIME: 4 MINUTES

- Lying on your side, bend your knees, so the soles of your feet are in a line with your spine
- Slowly lift the top knee up in an arc away from the other knee
- Hold for 3 seconds and then return slowly to resting
- Repeat 15 times x 3.

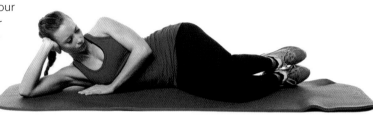

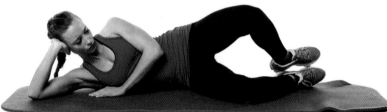

Hip flexors

(STRETCH) TIME: 1.5 MINUTES

- Stand in a forward lunge position
- Knee onto a cushion, if more comfortable
- Keep the torso upright
- Tuck your glutes under your pelvis

- Slowly bend the front knee so the stretch on the front of your hip increases
- Hold at a comfortable stretch for 45 seconds.

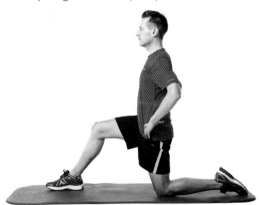

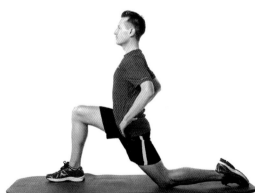

Hip Adductors

(STRETCH) TIME: 1.5 MINUTES

- Lunge to the side, bending your leading leg and keeping the trail leg straight
- Keep the pelvis level
- Slowly increase the bend in the lead leg until you reach a comfortable stretch on the inner side of the trail leg.
- Hold for 45 seconds.

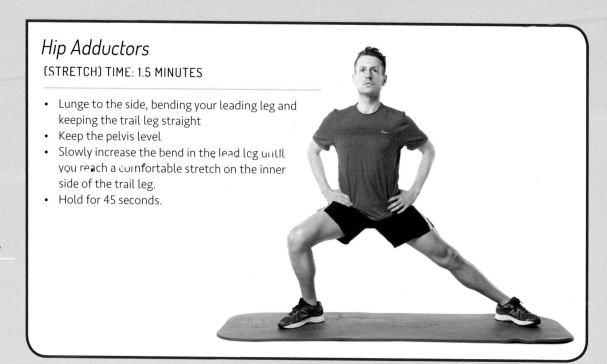

Hamstrings

(STRENGTH) TIME: 4 MINUTES

The use of this exercise as an eccentric muscle contraction requires the movements to be slow and controlled, lowering over approximately 6 seconds and back up at a controlled 1–2 second pace.

- From standing on one leg, slightly bend the supporting leg
- Bend forwards very slowly, whilst keeping the free leg straight
- Lower hands towards the floor, stop at the feeling of light stretch
- Return slowly to standing
- Alternate each leg
- Repeat 15 times each leg.

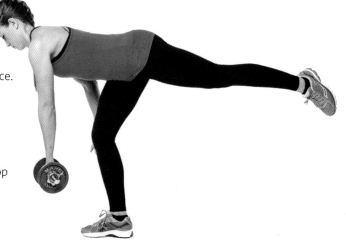

Single leg squat

(STRENGTH) TIME: 2 MINUTES

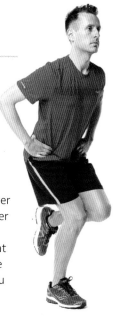

- Keep the knee over the middle toe
- Lower down as far as you can without the knee moving into the midline
- As soon as you see the knee disappearing over towards the big toe side, stop and come back up again
- Resist the temptation to move into a deeper squat until you can control the medial movement.

Start with 10 reps each side to begin with, developing the number of reps over the week rather than the depth of the squat. Each week drop 5–10cms deeper into the squat and reduce the reps initially, then build these up as the week progresses. This way you will only be increasing the difficulty of one aspect at a time. Within a matter of weeks you will notice that you can hold your knee plumb straight and get your knee bend below 90 degrees, way past what you need for running.

Glute activation

(STRENGTH) TIME: 4 MINUTES

This strengthens the core muscles by incorporating three exercises: the plank, glute activation and shoulder stabilization.

- Lie on your front
- Bend one knee to 90 degrees
- Imagine there is a tray of glasses on the sole of the raised foot
- Hold your foot very steady, careful not to change the knee bend
- Lift the leg upward using the glute only
- Slowly return the leg back down
- Repeat 5 times with a bent knee and once with a straight leg x 5
- Make this exercise harder by starting in the plank position instead.

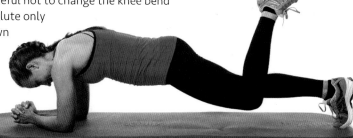

Core muscles

(STRENGTH) TIME: 3 MINUTES

- Lie on your back, legs bent at 90 degrees
- Place your fingertips onto the bony points at the front of the pelvis (anterior superior iliac spine (ASIS)) as shown
- Move your fingers in and down 2cm so you are pushing gently down on the transverse abdominis (TA) muscle
- You can check you are in the right place by coughing: you should feel the muscle bounce under your fingertips
- Relocate if necessary until this happens
- Imagine you are urinating and that you now stop the flow, you should feel a tightening of the TA. Hold that tension
- Draw in your belly button
- Slightly flatten your lower back toward the floor
- Hold all three of these positions together and you have tensed your core muscles accurately.

To test how strong your core is, alternate lifting each foot off the floor slightly, maintaining the tension equally in both sides of your TA muscle. When you can hold these both solid for 25 reps of each leg, you have activated your transverse abdominals and therefore your core, and you are ready to move onto more challenging exercises.

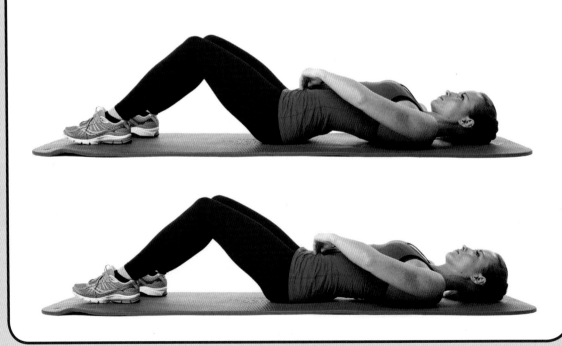

Hamstring/core combination
(STRENGTH) TIME: 1.5 MINUTES

This exercise includes the hamstring curl, bridge, and core activation in one.

- Lie on the floor with your heels resting on a fitness ball
- Engage the core as per the previous exercise
- Pull heels towards you and raise hips at the same time
- Release back to flat under control
- Repeat 8–10 reps x 3.

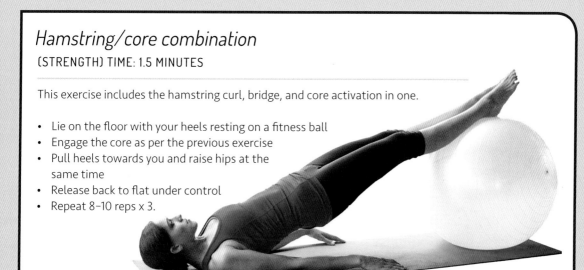

Glutes
(STRETCH) TIME: 1.5 MINUTES

- Sit on a chair, bringing one leg on top of the other knee
- Lean forwards until you feel a stretch in the glutes
- To increase the stretch, lift the heel from the floor
- Hold each stretch for 45–60 seconds.

FOR THE FLOOR STRETCH
- Lie on the ground
- With your left hand take hold of your left knee
- With your right hand, take hold of the left ankle using an under-hand grip
- Pull both towards you until you feel a stretch in the glutes
- Hold for 45–60 seconds.

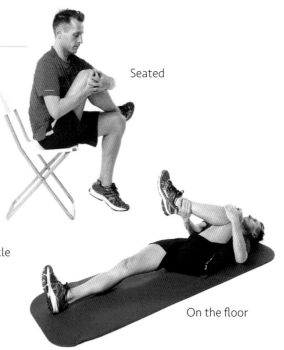

Seated

On the floor

Hamstring

(STRETCH) TIME: 1.5 MINUTES

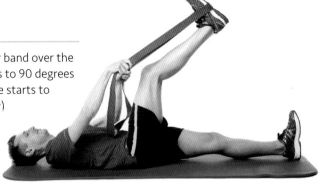

- Pull your leg towards you with a belt or band over the heel of your foot so that your hip flexes to 90 degrees
- Now pull on the band so that your knee starts to straighten (but doesn't straighten fully)
- Pull just enough so that you feel a good (but not really painful) stretch in the back of your upper leg
- Hold for 45 seconds.

Using a straight leg, which was the old fashioned method for the hamstring stretch, often stresses the sciatic nerve rather than the muscle, and pain is felt at the back of the knee instead.

Tensor fascia latae

(STRETCH) TIME: 1.5 MINUTES

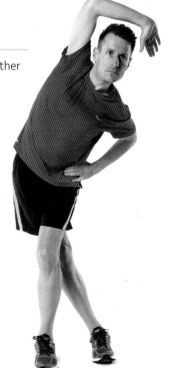

- Stand with one leg all the way around the back of the other
- Side bend to the side of the back foot
- Push the hip into the stretch
- Hold for 30–40 seconds.

Side step with squat

(STRENGTH) TIME: 4 MINUTES

This exercise activates the quads, glutes, abductors, adductors, calf, peroneal, and core muscles.

- Place a band around your thighs just tight enough to be put on a stretch when you bend your knees into a squat. Each rep contains three parts:
  - Squat
  - Side step
  - Return to standing
- Repeat this for the length of your available space or 10 reps each direction x 3.

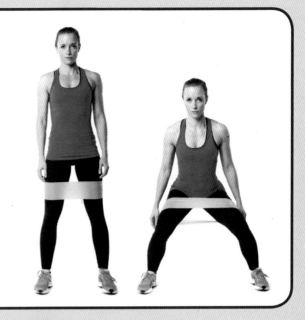

Eccentric calf raises

Eccentric loading is where you only stress the muscle on the return against gravity or resistance.

- Start on tiptoes
- Stand on one leg (the leg to be exercised eccentrically)
- Slowly lower the heel to the end of your available ankle range
- Place the free foot back onto the step
- Remove the injured leg
- Push back to the start position with the good leg
- Change feet again and repeat the process
- 3 x 15 reps on alternate days. Take 6 seconds from tiptoes to end of range
- Add weight via a rucksack or at the gym to ensure the loading is near maximal for the 3 x 15 reps.

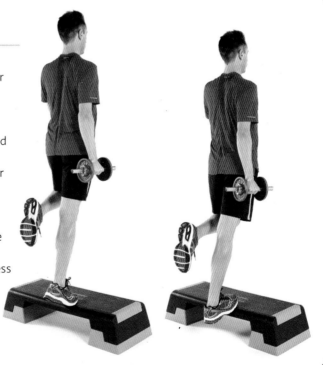

Sciatic nerve flossing

- Sit on a bench or table top
- Slump down slightly and nod your head forwards
- Start to straighten your leg at the knee until you feel tension then point your toes and hold for 5 seconds
- Now only moving your neck and ankle, raise the toes and the head at the same time and again hold for 5 seconds
- Repeat approximately 25 times, 2 or 3 sets per day.

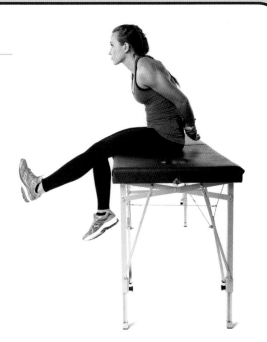

Swiss ball abduction in side plank

- Lie on your side on a gym ball and hold a side plank
- Lift the top leg up into abduction
- Hold for 3 seconds and slowly lower
- Repeat 15 times for each leg.

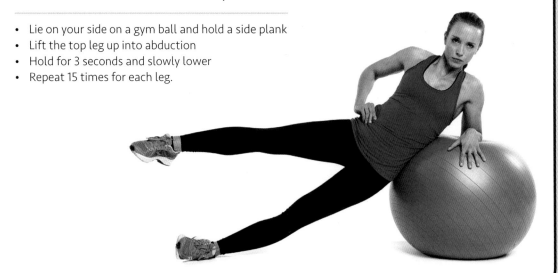

Inner range quad

- Roll up a towel and place it under your knee
- Press down with the back of your knee into the towel
- Your foot should start to move off the floor
- Tense the quadriceps around the knee as the foot is lifted until the leg is straight
- Bring the toes up to tighten the contraction around the knee
- Slowly lower back down
- Repeat 3 x 15 reps.

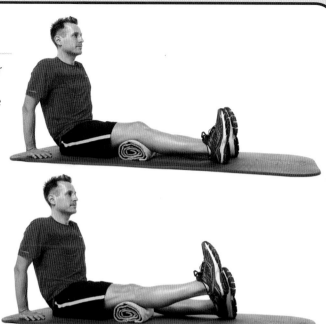

Quads foam rolling

- Lay on your front and place a foam roller under your upper thigh
- Place the free leg crossed over the back of the working leg
- Roll up towards your head, so the roller moves down along the thigh towards the knee
- Stop just before the knee, reset back to the start position without load and repeat 10 times.

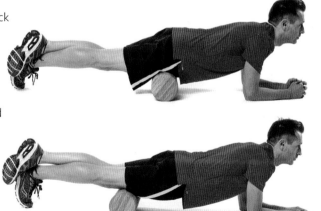

Quads stretch

- Stand facing a wall, balance yourself with one hand
- Use the other hand to pull up the leg to be stretched by the ankle
- Hold this for 45 seconds
- Change the hold so you are grasping the foot on the big toe side, pull outward to the side and repeat the 45-second hold
- Change the hold again by grasping the little toe side of the foot and pulling your foot into the opposite glute and hold for a further 45 seconds.

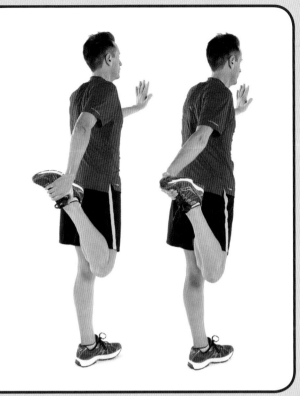

Hamstring curl (eccentric contraction)

- With a partner, and using some exercise band, lay flat on a mat
- Your partner should wrap the band around your ankle, allowing you to bend your knee without resistance
- Resist the band's tension whilst slowly extending the knee, thus making your hamstrings work against the resistance. This will ensure that you are using the hamstring muscles eccentrically, as prescribed
- Complete 3 x 15 reps.

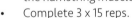

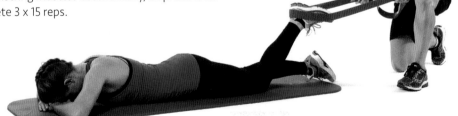

Nordic hamstring curls

- You need a friend to help you by holding your ankles
- Start with your knee at 90 degrees (kneeling)
- Slowly lower your body forward, careful to keep straight
- Work your core to ensure you keep straight between your knees and shoulders
- Only go as far as you can manage to hold the technique
- At first move forwards just a few inches
- Build up the distance you travel over a period of weeks
- Move as slowly as possible on the way down
- 3 x 10 reps on alternate days.

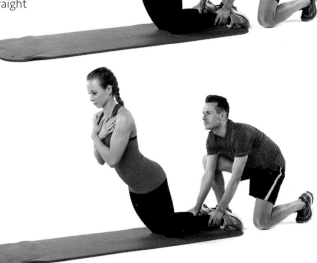

Piriformis stretch

- Lie on your front
- Pull the leg to be stretched underneath your torso
- Spread the foot out to the opposite side of your body
- Place your hands on the floor
- Lean forwards into the stretch
- The stretch will be felt deep inside the glute on that side
- Hold for 45 seconds and repeat 3 times.

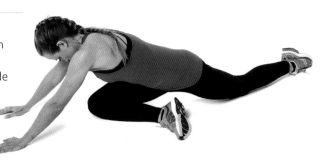

McKenzie back extensions

- Lie on your front
- Place your hands under your shoulders
- Lift up your head and shoulders
- Keep your legs relaxed
- Lower back down again
- Continue if pain does not spread into the glutes or legs
- If the pain centralizes (becomes more apparent in one spot within your back) you may continue cautiously, but not if the pain spreads
- Start with 3 x 10 repetitions but quickly build the number of reps as your pain allows.

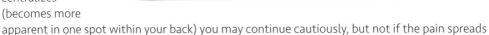

Eventually, you can stop using your arms for support and make this into more of a strength exercise by using the muscles in your lower back to lift your head and shoulders up rather than your arms pushing you up.

Bridge

- Lie on your back and bend your knees to 90 degrees
- Feet flat on the floor
- Engage your core muscles (see Core muscles, page 176)
- Lift your hips off the floor and hold in a line between shoulders and knees
- Hold for 10 seconds and slowly lower back down
- Repeat 10 times.

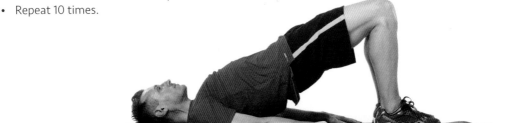

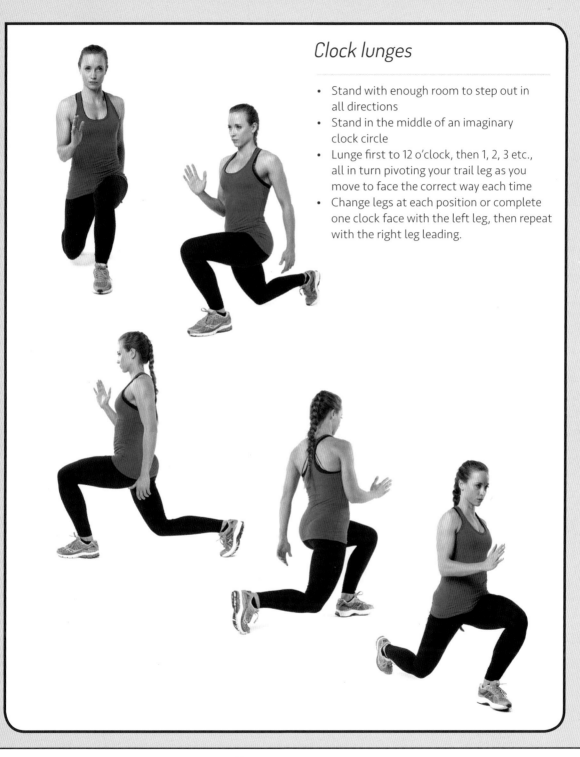

Clock lunges

- Stand with enough room to step out in all directions
- Stand in the middle of an imaginary clock circle
- Lunge first to 12 o'clock, then 1, 2, 3 etc., all in turn pivoting your trail leg as you move to face the correct way each time
- Change legs at each position or complete one clock face with the left leg, then repeat with the right leg leading.

Multi-direction hopping

- Stand on one leg
- Hop forwards and land on a bent knee
- Hop backwards to the start position
- Hop to the left then back to the centre again
- Hop to the right and back to centre again
- Hop backwards and then to the centre again
- Continue to hop in a variety of directions, including diagonals, in no particular pattern.

You do not need to always come back to the centre. If you have room, travel in all directions.

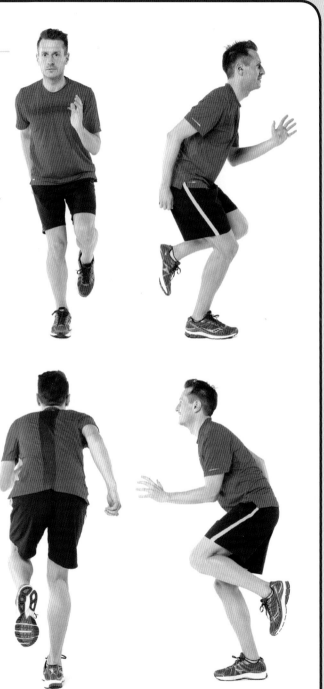

APPENDIX 2

WARM-UP AND COOL DOWN

Warm-Up

Warming up is thought to reduce muscle injury and to reduce stiffness related to prior muscle fatigue or injury. Unfortunately a high percentage of people walk out of the door, jog for 30 seconds before getting into their run, and return home for a rushed shower before heading out to work. This is a false economy, as you save time on that given day, but lose many weeks through injury further down the line. For those of you reading this claiming to have never been injured using this method of 'just running' then consider how your performances have improved (or not) in recent months. Unless you are new to running, it's highly likely that your

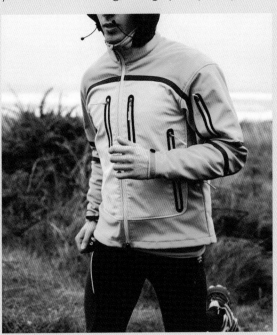

performance has plateaued, your PB for most distances occurred at least a year ago and your training programme lacks progression.

However, the warm up outlined below only takes several minutes to complete. In some cases this will be as long or longer than your intended run, so we have to be realistic. It is unlikely that I am going to change your lifelong habits and get you warming up for 20-25 minutes before a 30-minute run. However, read on, see what is 'gold standard' and then at the end of this section, see if my 'RRP' (rapid runners prep.) is a compromise when the full set cannot be completed due to time commitments.

FULL WARM-UP

Start with some gentle exercise such as 5-10 minutes on a bike, cross trainer or gentle jog, aimed at increasing blood flow, body temperature and therefore local muscle temperature. This phase of the warm-up will increase the heart rate gently, preparing the whole body for the planned exercise and also the mobility phase of the warm-up.

The second stage is to develop muscle length. Unlike the pre-habilitation exercises that use a lot of static stretching, this is a time to use dynamic stretches, or stretches through increased movement patterns.

Dynamic exercises such as high knees, heel-to-bum flicks, side stepping, and step cross overs all serve to gradually increase the length of the muscle through movement, however these individual movements can be efficiently done across just two exercises and their variations.

The comprehensive runners' warm-up is shown below.

Multi-direction lunge

- Start with mini lunges in all directions. The movement needs to start small and build in depth, so the muscles get used to the movement
- Build the depth slightly each lunge and gradually allow the muscles to warm up
- Lunge forwards, backwards, to the side and then start to add a small twist, building the twist again with each repetition.
- You should aim to achieve over 20 reps with each leg.

NB: The full lunge with twist stretches just about every muscle required for running, even the contractile element of the ITB is gaining length here.

Pendulum legs

- After the lunges, move to leg swings in all directions
- Imagine your leg is a pendulum, swinging back and forth, slowly and with a short range at first, building in height and rhythm as your muscle allows
- Try not to force it
- Now move out to the side and back across the midline, in front and behind the standing leg.

NB: keep a (slightly) bent knee throughout the exercise, gradually building the range of movement as the exercise develops over 20–30 repetitions in each direction.

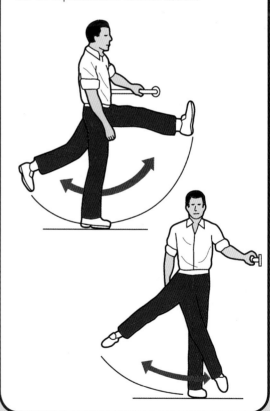

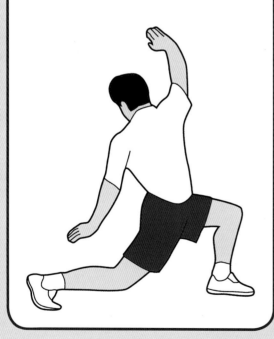

RRP – the rapid runners' preparation – 9½ minutes

- Jog very slowly for 2 minutes – no build in pace
- Jog at a medium pace for 2 minutes – no build in pace
- Lunge walk x 12 steps (each leg) forwards, first lunge mini dip, building to 12th lunge as a full movement.
- Side lunge x 12 steps (each leg), build depth from 1-12
- Reverse lunge x 12 steps, as above
- Jog medium pace for 2 minutes
- Twist lunge x 12 as above
- Leg swings x 12 in each direction, building distance from 1–12
- Jog for 1 minute at a steady pace to finish warm-up.

Cool down

The cool down is as important for your cardiovascular system as it is for your muscles themselves. You should gradually cool down over 5 minutes as a minimum, allowing the heart rate to gradually lower. After this static stretching can be a real benefit, but not performed aggressively, see this as a chance to restore range of movement rather than as the key time for development. Regular stretching throughout the day is a great time to hold the stretches for longer and work on development of length.

I want to quickly look at some potential myths associated with stretching. Yes there has been research to show that some runners had a loss of performance directly following static stretching, but none of the tested athletes had any performance reduction following dynamic stretching – hence the use of dynamic stretching just before exercise. It is important to note that static stretching still has its place and these few studies showing a reduction in performance are in no way suggesting we abandon static stretching at other times. Secondly, it is highly unlikely that going for a standard training run will be negatively affected by whichever type of stretching you choose and this shouldn't create a 'throwing the baby out with the bath water' approach to this new information. Lastly, if you are currently injured, then you will potentially (and highly likely) have a chronic muscle shortening, which needs specific attention. Performing your rehabilitation exercises for muscle length prior to a rehab or early training run is not only fine, its important for your return to full fitness. I advocate any potential loss in performance for these runs, in favour of injury protection.

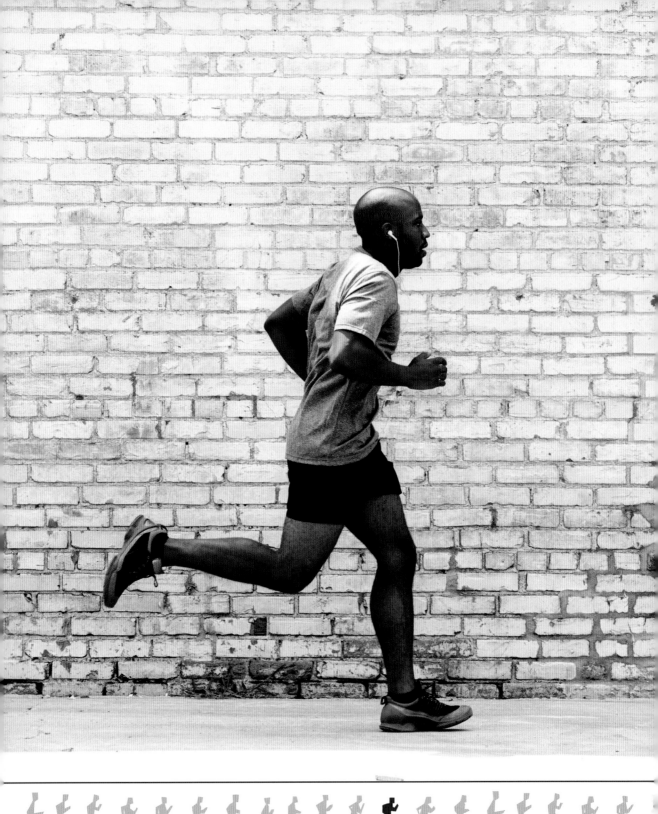

TRAINING PLANS

5k running programme – 7 weeks from beginner to 5k

Week	Mon	Tue	Wed	Thur	Fri	Sat	Sun
1	Rest	1min jog 2min walk x 10	Rest	4min jog 1min rest x 4	Rest	1km jog 3min rest x 2	Rest
2	Rest	1min jog 2min walk x 10	Rest	4min jog 1min rest x 4	Rest	1km jog 2min rest x 2	Rest
3	Rest	1min jog 2min walk x 12	Rest	4min jog 1min rest x 5	Rest	1km jog 2min rest x 3	Rest
4	Rest	Rest	Rest	4min jog 1min rest x 5	Rest	1km jog 1min rest x 3	Rest
5	Rest	1min jog 2min walk x 14	Rest	4min jog 1min rest x 6	Rest	1km jog 2min rest x 4	Rest
6	Rest	2min jog 1min walk x 8	Rest	4min run 2min rest x 4	Rest	1km run 3min jog x 4	Rest
7	Rest	Rest	Rest	4min run 1min rest x 4	Rest	Rest	5k jog

5k running programme – 7 weeks *intermediate* in search of a PB

Week	Mon	Tue	Wed	Thur	Fri	Sat	Sun
1	Rest	4min threshold 3min recovery x 4	Rest	Hill reps 30 sec hill Max effort x 12 Walk back Recovery	Rest	60min tempo run	Rest
2	Rest	4min threshold 3min recovery x 5	Rest	40min tempo	Rest	1km reps x 4 PB pace – 10 sec	Rest
3	Rest	4min threshold 3min recovery x 6	Rest	Hill reps 30 sec hill Max effort x 12 Walk back Recovery	Rest	70min tempo run	Rest
4	Rest	3min threshold 2min recovery x 8	Rest	60min tempo	Rest	1km reps x 5 PB pace – 15 sec	Rest
5	Rest	3min threshold 2min recovery x 10	Rest	Hill reps 30 sec hill Max effort x 12 Walk back Recovery	Rest	80min tempo run	Rest
6	Rest	2min threshold 1min recovery x 12	Rest	30min sub-race pace	Rest	1km reps x 6 PB pace – 5 sec	Rest
7	5k recovery jog	Rest	Rest	25min jog	Rest	Rest	5km time trial

10k running programme – 7 weeks *intermediate* in search of a PB

Week	Mon	Tue	Wed	Thur	Fri	Sat	Sun
1	30min run	10 x 1min on, 1min off (jog) in the middle of a 5 mile run	20min jog	5 mile tempo, feeling relaxed	20min light jog	10 x 1min hills	8 mile run
2	30min run	5 x 1km off (jog) 2min recovery	20min light jog	4 mile tempo	Rest	5km race	8 mile run
3	30min run	10 x 400m off (jog) 60 seconds recovery, race pace	Rest	6 mile tempo	20min run	10 x 1min hills	10 mile run
4	30min run	6 x 1 mile off (jog) 2min recovery	20min jog	4 mile tempo	20min run	10 x 1min hills	10 mile run
5	30min run	10 x 1min on, 1min off (jog) in the middle of a 5 mile run	Rest	4 mile tempo plus 3 x 60 seconds FAST at the end	Rest	5k race	8 mile run
6	30min run	10 x 400m off (jog) 60 seconds recovery, race pace	20min jog	6 mile tempo	20min run	3 miles at race pace	8 mile run
7	30min run	10 x 1min on, 1min off (jog) in the middle of a 5 mile run	Rest	3 mile tempo	20min nice and easy	10km race	Rest

TRAINING PLANS

10k running programme – 8 weeks **advanced** in search of a PB

Week	Mon	Tue	Wed	Thur	Fri	Sat	Sun
1	8 mile run with strides	10 x 1min on, 1min off (jog) in the middle of a 10 mile run	45mins	10 miles	8 mile tempo feeling relaxed	30mins easy	15 mile long run nice and steady
2	8 mile run	4 x 5 x 400m – 3min between sets and 200m slow jog recovery between reps. Race pace and getting quicker	45min run relaxed to recover	10 miles with strides	4 x 2 miles with 5min recovery. Lots of recovery so these need to be quick	30min nice and easy	18 mile long run
3	8 mile run with strides	3 x 8 x 60 seconds on / 60 seconds off (jog) with a long warm up and long warm down	Rest	2 x 5 x 200m 400m jog recovery between sets and 200m jog between reps fast	30min nice and easy	5k race (maybe a park run)	15 mile long run
4	8 mile run	10 x 400m with 60 seconds recovery. At race pace and quicker	45min run	30min nice and easy with strides	5 x 1 mile with 2:30min recovery – on a path/grass	10 miles nice and easy	15 mile long run
5	Rest	6 mile tempo and then 3 x 60 seconds fast (race pace)	30min run	10 mile run	10 x 1min on, 1min off (jog) in the middle of a 10 mile run	30min nice and easy or rest	15 mile long run

Week	Mon	Tue	Wed	Thur	Fri	Sat	Sun
6	8 mile run	8 x 1km at race pace with 3min recovery. Perhaps start with 2 x 200m to loosen up	45min run	2 x 5 x 200m. 400m jog recovery between sets and 200m jog between reps. FAST	30min run	5k race (maybe a park run)	15 mile long run
7	8 mile run	2 x 5 x 1km first 5 off, 60 sec recovery and second 5 off, 75 sec recovery	30min easy	8 mile run	3 x 15min efforts with 5min recovery	30min easy	12 mile long run
8	Rest	10 x 400m with 60 seconds recovery. At race pace and quicker	30min easy	2 x 5 x 200m. 400m jog recovery between sets and 200m jog between reps. FAST	20min light jog with strides	10k race	Rest

Marathon running programme – 12 weeks *beginner* in search of a PB

Week	Mon	Tue	Wed	Thur	Fri	Sat	Sun
1	20min run	30min run	40min run	Rest	60min run with 5 x 1min hard efforts in the middle	30min run	10 miles
2	30min light jog	5 x 1k efforts with 3min recovery	45min run	6 mile tempo getting quicker as it goes on. Starting off slower than race pace	Rest	5k park run with 30min afterwards	13 miles
3	30min run	5 x 1 mile with 90sec recovery	30min run	60mins	20min light jog with strides	10k race or race pace	
4	20min light jog	45min run	5 x 10min efforts with 4min recovery	20min light jog	8 mile tempo around race pace or a little slower	30min light jog	15 miles
5	30min run	10 x 1km off 60sec	20min light jog	60min run	8 mile tempo around race pace or a little slower	30min light jog	18 miles
6	30min run	10 x 1min on and 1min off (jog) recovery with warm up and warm down	50min run	30min light jog	10 mile tempo averaging 10sec per mile slower than race pace	Rest	20 miles

Week	Mon	Tue	Wed	Thur	Fri	Sat	Sun
7	30min light jog	10 x 400m off 45sec recovery. Start at race pace and work down	90min run	30min light jog	8 mile tempo averaging 10sec per mile slower than race pace	Rest	20 miles
8	60min light jog	2 x 5 x 3mins with 1min recovery and 3min between sets	45min run	Rest	12 mile tempo averaging 10sec per mile slower than race pace	Rest	18 miles
9	30min light jog	2 mile at race pace, 3min recovery, 10 x 800m off, 60secs recovery. 3min recovery then 2 mile at race pace again	45min run	30min light jog	30min light jog	10k race or 10 mile run	
10	30min light jog	15min tempo at race pace. 3min recovery and then 5 x 1 mile quicker than race pace with 1min recovery	10 mile run	60–75min run	5 mile tempo race pace or quicker	Rest	18 miles
11	60min run	4 x 2 miles with 4min recovery. Start at quicker than race pace and work down.	10 mile run	60min run	8 mile tempo averaging 10sec per mile slower than race pace	60min run	10 mile run
12	45min nice and easy with strides	12 x 3mins with a 2min recovery	30mins nice and easy	30min light jog and strides	Rest	20min light jog	Marathon race

* This is still quite a bit of running, but in order to get round a marathon you are going to need to do some running! In this programme the athlete isn't going to be running as far in the long run and slightly less in the tempos. I still think the long runs are important, if you like take out some of the steady runs in between the sessions – they are not as important. You'd have a better handle on what kind of level you are targeting with these guys.

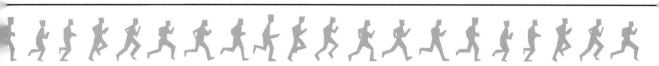

Marathon running programme – 12 weeks **advanced** in search of a PB

Week	Mon	Tue	Wed	Thur	Fri	Sat	Sun
1	Rest	5 x 1km off, 1min recovery	30min run	45min run	5 x 2km at race pace off 3min recovery	45min run	14 miles
2	30min light jog	5 x 1mile at 20 seconds quicker per mile than race pace (90 seconds recovery)	90min run	Rest	8 mile tempo getting quicker as it goes on. Starting off slower than race pace	30min run	16 miles
3	60min run	(3km, 2km, 1km) x 2 all off 3min recovery. All quicker than race pace	30min run	60mins	20min light jog	10km race or race effort this weekend	
4	45min run	4 x 12min runs that include 2 hills	90min run	Rest	8 mile tempo around race pace or a little slower	45min light jog	20 miles
5	60min run	10 x 1km off 60 seconds	75min run	60min run	2 x 5miles off 6min recovery	30min light jog	20 miles
6	45min run	75min run	60min run	30min light jog	10 mile tempo averaging 10 sec per mile slower than race pace	Rest	22 miles

Week	Mon	Tue	Wed	Thur	Fri	Sat	Sun
7	30min light jog	15 x 400m off, 45 seconds recovery. Start at race pace and work down	90min run	30min light jog	12 mile tempo averaging 10 sec per mile slower than race pace	Rest	24 miles
8	60min light jog	2 x 5 x 3mins with 1min recovery and 3min between sets	75min run	30min light jog	14 mile tempo averaging 10sec per mile slower than race pace	45min run easy	20 miles
9	30min light jog	2 mile at race pace. 3min recovery 10 x 800m off, 60 secs recovery. 3min recovery then 2 mile at race pace again	75min run	60min light jog	30min light jog	10km race or 10 mile run (not a half marathon)	
10	60min run	15min tempo at race pace. 3min recovery and then 5 x 1 mile quicker than race pace with 1min recovery	14 mile run	60–75min run	5 mile tempo race pace or quicker	Rest	20 miles
11	60min run	4 x 2 miles with 4min recovery. Start at quicker than race pace and work down	14 mile run	60min run	Tempo – 10 miles, target just slower than race pace	60min run	14 mile run
12	60min nice and easy + strides	12 x 3mins with a 2min recovery	45mins nice and easy	50min light jog + strides	Rest	20min light jog	Marathon race

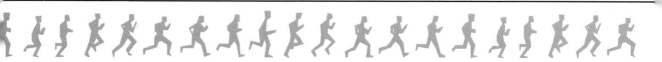

FINAL COMMENTS

What this book has attempted to provide every runner of any ability with is an insight into the types of injuries that can be sustained and what you can do yourself to both recognize them and to develop early management strategies whilst you wait for a physiotherapy appointment.

It was my intention that you would keep this on your bookshelf and reach for it whenever you felt a niggle to see what you would do with respect to rest, continuing to train or to seeking professional help.

It is not my intention however that you consult this book in an attempt to avoid ever seeking help again, or consider yourself a trained professional. I feel that there is enough information here to assist a runner in taking control of his or her injury, to question the therapists he or she may meet, but not to use the information garnered as a stick to beat them.

I also hope that some physiotherapists and other professionals will consider this book helpful in their management of their clients' injuries, opening up debate on what, for example, is the best practice for runner's knee, or whether the sacroiliac joint actually moves. I sincerely hope that we are getting to a point within the health care services where we can start to agree with each other and do what's right for the client.

I hope that the students of various healthcare courses can dip into the book and take some useful information from it, but I do have to warn you this is not an academic text and is full of my own thoughts and ideas.

I also really hope that you enjoyed reading about my clients' journeys. I asked them all to write down, in their own words, what their experience had been through their injury. This gives you a chance to see that someone else has been through the same injury as you, and that it is something that you can conquer. In some cases, the stories have shown the person go beyond the injury and actually become a better runner, suggesting perhaps that the pending and building injury was in some way holding them back, or, more likely I believe, that they finally did some strength and conditioning work, which resulted in a stronger core with more flexible extremities.

This book will not cure injuries, it won't take your pain away simply by reading it, but it will make you a better runner, it will make you more informed and prevent you having to rely on the old timer at your club who appears to be the font of all knowledge (sorry if that's you).

Good luck to all of you!

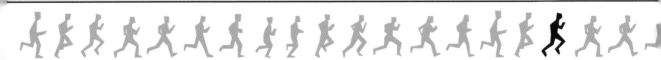

BIBLIOGRAPHY

Baker, K.G., Robertson, V., Duck, F. (2001) 'A Review of Therapeutic Ultrasound: Biophysical Effects', *Physical Therapy*, 81(7), pp.1351–58.

Baltich, J. *et al.* (2015) 'The Influence of Ankle Strength Exercise Training on Running Injury Risk Factors', *Footwear Science*, 7(sup1).

Blackman, P.G. (2000) 'A review of chronic exertional compartment syndrome in the lower leg' *Medicine and Science in Sports and Exercise*, 32(3) s.4-10.

Cacchio, A. *et al.* (2011) 'Shockwave Therapy for the Treatment of Chronic Proximal Hamstring Tendinopathy in Professional Athletes', *American Journal of Sports Medicine*, 39(1), pp.146–53.

Campbell, J. T. (2009) 'Posterior Calf Injury; Foot and Ankle Clinics', *Foot Ankle Clin.*, 14(4), pp.761–71.

Carter, D. (2015) 'Analgesia for people with acute ankle sprain. Literature review on using non-steroidal anti-inflammatory drugs in the management of a common injury', *Emergency Nurse*, 23(1), pp.24–31.

Chuter, V.H., Xanne, A.K., de Jonge, J. (2012) 'Proximal and distal contributions to lower extremity injury: A review of the literature', *Gait & Posture*, 36(1) pp.7–15.

Christina, C., White, S., Gilchrist, L. (2001) 'Effect of localized muscle fatigue on vertical ground reaction forces and ankle joint motion during running', *Human Movement Science*, 20(3), pp.257–76.

Czyzewski, A. (2012) 'Shin splints most common musculoskeletal injury in runners', *Sports Med.* 2(42), pp.891–905.

Dias Lopes, A., Hespanhol, L.C., Yeung, S., Pena Costa, L.O. (2012) 'What are the Main Running-Related Musculoskeletal Injuries?', *Systematic Review: Sports Medicine*, 42(10), pp.891–905.

Fallon, K., Purdam, C., Cook, J., Lovell, G. (2008) 'A Polypill for acute tendon pain in athletes with tendinopathy?', *Journal of Science and Medicine in Sport, Elsevier Opinion Piece*, 11, pp.235–38.

Feinstein, B. *et al.* (1955) 'Morphologic Studies of Motor Units in Normal Human Muscles', *Acta Anatomica*, 23(2), pp.127-42.

Hall, C., and Nester, C.J. (2004) 'Sagittal Plane Compensations for Artificially Induced Limitation of the First Metatarsophalangeal Joint: A Preliminary Study', *Journal of Applied Podiatric Medical Association*, 94(3), pp.269–74.

Hamstra-Wright, K.L., Huxel-Bliven, K.C.,Bay. C. (2015) 'Risk factors for medial tibial stress syndrome in physically active individuals such as runners and military personnel: a systematic review and meta-analysis', *Br. J. Sports Med.* 49, pp.362–69.

Hardy, R.H., Clapham, J.C.R. (1952) 'Valgus Predisposing Anatomical Causes', Department of Anatomy, University College London, UK. 259(6720) pp.1180–83.

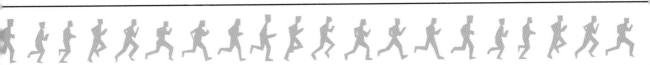

Hawker, G.A., Mian, A., Kendzerska, T. and French, M. (2011) 'Measures of adult pain: Visual Analog Scale for Pain (VAS Pain), Numeric Rating Scale for Pain (NRS Pain), McGill Pain Questionnaire (MPQ), Short-Form McGill Pain Questionnaire (SF-MPQ), Chronic Pain Grade Scale (CPGS), Short Form-36 Bodily Pain Scale (SF-36 BPS), and Measure of Intermittent and Constant Osteoarthritis Pain (ICOAP)', *Arthritis Care & Research*. 63(11) pp.S240–S252.

Hertel, J. (2000) 'Functional Instability Following Lateral Ankle Sprain', *Sports Medicine*, 29(5), pp.361–71.

Hiemstra, L.A., Webber, S., MacDonald, P.B., Kriellaars, D.J. (2007). 'Contralateral limb strength deficits after anterior cruciate ligament reconstruction using a hamstring tendon graft.' *Clinical Biomechanics*. 22(5), pp.543–550.

Hill, J., Howartson, G., Van Someren, K., Walshe, I., Pedlar, C. (2014) 'Influence of compression garments on recovery after marathon running', *Journal of Strength and Conditioning Research*. 28(8), pp.2228–35.

Jansen and Kamper (2013) 'Ankle taping and bracing for proprioception', *Br. J. Sports Med.* 47, pp.527–28.

Jones, P. *et al.* (2015) 'Oral non-steroidal anti-inflammatory drugs versus other oral analgesic agents for acute soft tissue injury', *Cochrane Database of Systematic Reviews*, 7.

Karlsson, J. and Andreasson, G.O. (1992) 'The effect of external ankle support in chronic lateral ankle joint instability: An electromyographic study.' *Am. J. Sports Med*, 20(3) pp.257–61.

Kreamer, W.J. *et al.* (2001) 'Influence of compression therapy on symptoms following soft tissue injury following maximal eccentric exercises', *Journal of Orthopaedic & Sports Physical Therapy*, 31(6), pp.282–90.

Kruse, L.M. (2012) 'Rehabilitation After Anterior Cruciate Ligament Reconstruction, A Systematic Review', *J. Bone Joint Surg. Am.*, 94(19), pp.1737–48.

Kulmala, J. *et al.* (2013) 'Forefoot Strikers Exhibit Lower Running-Induced Knee Loading than Rearfoot Strikers' *Medicine and Science in Sports and Exercise,* 45(12), pp.2306–13.

Lieberman, D. E. *et al.* (2010) 'Foot strike patterns and collision forces in habitually barefoot versus shod runners', *Nature*, 463, pp.531–35/ doi:10.1038.

Lustenberger, D.P., *et al.* (2013) 'Efficacy of Treatment of Trochanteric Bursitis: A Systematic Review', *Clin. J. Sport Med.*, 21(5), pp.447–53.

Macfarlane, G.J., Croft, T., Papageorgiou, P.R., Jayson, M.I., Silman, A.J. (1999) 'Predictors of early improvement in low back pain amongst consultants to general practice: the influence of pre-morbid and episode-related factors', 80(1–2), pp.113–119.

Malanga, G.A., Yan. N. and Stark, J. (2015) 'Mechanisms and efficacy of heat and cold therapies for musculoskeletal injury', *Postgraduate Medicine*, 127(1), pp.57–65.

Mani-Babu, S., *et al.* (2015) 'The Effectiveness of Extracorporeal Shock Wave Therapy in Lower Limb Tendinopathy – A Systematic Review', *Am. J. Sports Med.* 43(3), pp.752–61.

Matsuda, S. and Fukubayashi, T. (2015) *Sports Injuries and Prevention: Risk Factors and Mechanisms of Fifth Metatarsal Stress Fracture*, pp.355–36.

Myer, G.D. *et al.* (2005) 'Neuromuscular Training Improves Performance and Lower-Extremity Biomechanics in Female Athletes', *Journal of Strength and Conditioning Research,* 19(1): 51-60.

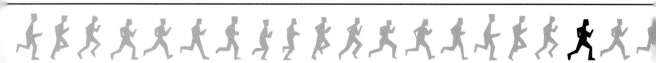

O'Leary, K., Anderson Vorpahl, K. and Heiderscheit, B. (2008) 'Effect of Cushioned Insoles on Impact Forces During Running', *Journal of the American Podiatric Medical Association*, 98(1), pp.36–41.

Piqué-Vidal, C., Solé, M. and Antich, J. (2007) 'Hallux Valgus Inheritance: Pedigree Research in 350 Patients With Bunion Deformity.' *Journal of Foot and Ankle Surgery*, 46(3), pp.149–154.

Rantanen, J. *et al.* (1999) 'Effects of Therapeutic Ultrasound on the Regeneration of Skeletal Myofibers After Experimental Muscle Injury', *Am. J. Sports Med.* 27(1), pp.54-59.

Riddle, D. L. *et al.* (2003) 'Risk Factors for Plantar Fasciitis: A Matched Case-Control Study', *Journal of Bone Joint Surg. Am.* 85(5): 872-877.

Ryan, W., Mahony, N., Delaney, M., O'Brien, M. and Murray P.,(2003) 'Relationship of the common peroneal nerve and its branches to the head and neck of the fibula', *Clinical Anatomy,* 16(6), pp.501–05.

Sihvonen, R. *et al.* (2013) 'Arthroscopic Partial Meniscectomy versus Sham Surgery for a Degenerative Meniscal Tear', *N. Engl. J. Med.,* 369, pp.2515–24.

Tiidus, P. M. (2015) 'Alternative treatments for muscle injury: massage, cryotherapy, and hyperbaric oxygen', *Current Reviews in Musculoskeletal Medicine*, 8(2), pp.162–67.

Tojima, M., Noma, K., Torii, S. (2015) 'Changes in serum creatine kinase, leg muscle tightness, and delayed onset muscle soreness after a full marathon race', *Journal of Sports Medicine and Physical Fitness*. E-Pub ahead of print.

Torres, R., Ribeiro, F., Duarte, J.A., Cabri, J. (2012). 'Evidence of the physiotherapeutic interventions used currently after exercise-induced muscle damage: Systematic review and meta-analysis', *Physical Therapy in Sport*, 13(2), pp.101–114.

Vleeming, A., Schuenke, M., Masi, A., Carreiro, J., Danneels, L. (2012) 'The sacroiliac joint: an overview of its anatomy, function and potential clinical implications', *J. Anat.* 221, pp.537–67.

Wang, C. (2012) 'Extracorporeal shockwave therapy in musculoskeletal disorders', *Journal of Orthopaedic Surgery and Research*, 7(11).

Warren, B. L. (1990) 'Sports Medicine; Plantar Fasciitis in Runners, Treatment and Prevention', 10(5), pp.38–345.

Wu, K. (1996) 'Morton's interdigital neuroma: A clinical review of its etiology, treatment, and results', *The Journal of Foot and Ankle Surgery*, 35(2), pp112–19.

INDEX

RUNNING FREE OF INJURIES

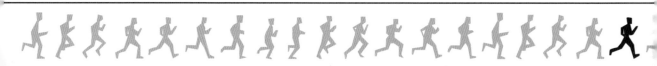

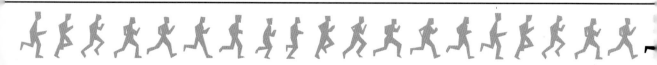